D1757390

About the Author

Susan Crocker Houde, PhD, APRN, BC, is Professor and Director of the Master's and Certificate Programs in Nursing at the University of Massachusetts, Lowell and is Associate Director of the Division of Aging of the Center for Health and Disease Research. She has a master's degree in gerontological nursing from the University of Lowell and a PhD in social policy with a specialty in aging from Brandeis University. Dr. Houde is certified as an adult nurse practitioner from ANCC. Dr. Houde is a Section Editor for Public Policy of the *Journal of Gerontological Nursing* and serves as a reviewer for several journals and professional organizations. She has published numerous articles and presented papers on issues related to aging and nursing care of the older adult. Her research interests include prevention of age-related vision loss, family caregiving of functionally impaired elders, and promotion of physical activity in older adults. She is a member of the Gerontological Society of America and the National Organization of Nurse Practitioner Faculties, where she serves on the Educational Standards and Guidelines Committee. Dr. Houde is a Research Scholar of the Hartford Institute of Geriatric Nursing.

Vision Loss in Older Adults

Nursing Assessment and Care Management

Edited by

SUSAN CROCKER HOUDE, PhD, APRN, BC

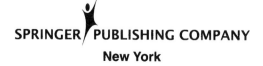

SPRINGER PUBLISHING COMPANY

New York

Springer Publishing Company, LLC
11 West 42nd Street
New York, NY 10036

Acquisitions Editor: Sally J. Barhydt
Production Editor: Peggy M. Rote
Cover Design: Joanne E. Honigman
Composition: Techbooks

07 08 09 10/5 4 3 2 1

Library of Congress Cataloging-in-Publication Data

Houde, Susan Crocker.
  Vision loss in older adults : nursing assessment and care management / Susan Crocker Houde.
      p. ; cm.
  Includes bibliographical references and index.
  ISBN-13: 978-0-8261-0218-8 (pbk.)
  ISBN-10: 0-8261-0218-2 (pbk.)
  1. Older people with visual disabilities–Care.   2. Older people with visual disabilities–Rehabilitation.   3. Adjustment (Psychology) in old age.   4. Geriatric nursing.   I. Houde, Susan Crocker.
  [DNLM: 1. Vision Disorders–nursing.   2. Aged.   3. Eye Diseases–nursing. WY 158 V834 2007]

RE48.2.A5V57 2007
618.97'77–dc22

        2006023071

Printed in the United States of America by Bang Printing.

Contents

Contributors

Pamela Z. Cacchione, PhD, RN, BC, GNP
Hartford Institute of Geriatric
Nursing Gerontological Research
Scholar
Associate Professor
School of Nursing, Doisy College of
Health Sciences
Saint Louis University
St. Louis, MO

Betsy Campochiaro, RN, MSN
Coordinator for the Macular
Degeneration Center
The Wilmer Eye Institute
Johns Hopkins University
Baltimore, MD

Pat Gillett, MSN, C-FNP, C-ACNP
Acute Care Nurse Practitioner
Concentration Coordinator
College of Nursing
University of New Mexico
Albuquerque, NM

Kate Goldblum, MSN, CS, FNP, CRNO
Goldblum Family Eye Care Center
Albuquerque, NM

Arlene McGrory, DNSc, RN
Associate Professor
Department of Nursing
University of Massachusetts
Lowell
Lowell, MA

Karen Devereaux Melillo, PhD, APRN, BC, FAANP
Professor and Chair
Department of Nursing
University of Massachusetts
Lowell
Lowell, MA

Judith M. Pentedemos, MS, APRN, BC, CDE
Joslin Clinic at Nashoba Valley
Medical Center
Ayer, MA

Joyce Powers, MSN, CS, FNP, ACNP, CS
Veterans Administration Medical
Center
Albuquerque, NM

Ruth Remington, PhD, APRN, BC
Assistant Professor
Department of Nursing
University of Massachusetts Lowell
Lowell, MA

Catherine S. Sackett, RN, CANP
The Wilmer Eye Institute
Johns Hopkins University
Baltimore, MD

Preface

Nurses play a vital role in the promotion of health and well-being of patients and in the support of family caregivers who provide care to functionally impaired older adults. Vision loss in older adults often leads to functional impairment and dependency. Nurses, with advanced knowledge of common vision problems in old age, can play an important role in education that may promote behaviors that can have a positive effect on preventing and slowing the progression of age-related vision loss. This is especially important because the prevalence of vision impairment due to age-related causes is expected to increase as the U.S. population ages. Globally, vision impairment is a major problem as well, with a high prevalence of blindness worldwide.

The four leading causes of age-related vision loss are (1) age-related macular degeneration, (2) cataracts, (3) glaucoma, and (4) diabetic retinopathy. This book provides professional nurses with information about these conditions, their causes, effects, diagnoses, and management. The signs, symptoms, and pathophysiology of these conditions will be discussed. Chapters on the psychological and social impact of vision loss and the issues faced by families of older adults with age-related vision loss will provide a foundation for nurses so that they can better meet the complex needs of individuals and families who are attempting to cope with the limitations that occur as a result of vision loss. Research is ongoing about strategies to prevent the occurrence and progression of age-related vision loss, especially in relation to age-related macular degeneration. Recent findings and suggestions for educating patients and families about preventing vision loss are also presented. Chapters on the care of older adults with vision loss as well as resources and information about new assistive devices will enable professional nurses to provide the comprehensive, quality nursing care that this population deserves and requires to maintain a high quality of life. The book concludes with some perspectives on future directions for care of older adults with vision loss.

It is my hope that this volume will be an important resource for practicing professional nurses who care for older adults and that it will encourage nurses to become more actively involved in meeting the multifaceted needs of older adults with vision problems and their families. Nurses, many of whom are in primary care roles, may be actively involved in the care of older adults with other chronic and acute health problems. Nurses may greatly enhance the comprehensive care of their older patients in all clinical settings by active involvement in enhancing eye health and facilitating adaptation to vision impairment.

I am pleased to have had the opportunity to edit this book on age-related vision problems in the older adult. At the age of 45, I was diagnosed with an age-related eye condition that has the potential for progressive vision loss, and the importance of compassionate support and education related to the eye condition was clearly evident. Despite my education as a gerontological nurse practitioner and my work in the nursing field for two decades, I found I had numerous questions and fears about the condition, the progression, and the impact the condition would have on my future functional ability. As I searched the nursing literature, I was alarmed to find that little was being written by nurses about vision loss. Seeking information about ways to prevent the progression of the disease and about available resources, I found vast literature available in other disciplines but very little in the field of nursing. Knowing of the lack of nursing resources and evidence-based findings, I proceeded to write several articles targeted for the gerontological nurse and the nurse practitioner based on my investigations. When Springer Publishing informed me that they were looking for someone to write a book about vision problems in older adults and asked if I would be willing to edit this book, I was thankful for the opportunity. I was also fortunate to find nurses who were knowledgeable about the topic area and willing to share their expertise with other nurses. In the past, care of patients with age-related vision problems was traditionally addressed by ophthalmologists. The nurse, however, is in an excellent position to detect, educate, refer, reinforce, identify resources, make recommendations, and support and inform patients and caregivers about recent developments in the prevention and treatment of age-related eye diseases. Nurses, patients, and family members should take an active role in seeking resources that are available for psychological and functional support. I hope this book will help nurses to feel more confident and competent in assuming an active role in the ophthalmic health care of their older adult patients.

Susan Crocker Houde, PhD, APRN, BC

Acknowledgments

There are many people I would like to acknowledge for providing me with the inspiration to complete this book. Springer Publishing Company recognized the importance for nurses in practice to have increased knowledge about vision problems in older adults. I appreciate both the opportunity they provided to edit this book and the assistance of the staff. I would also like to thank the chapter authors. The book would not have been possible without their contributions. They were willing to share their expertise, despite busy schedules, so that others could learn about this important area of health care for older adults.

I would also like to recognize Mathy Mezey and Amy Berman from the John A. Hartford Foundation Institute of Geriatric Nursing at New York University for assistance in identifying contributors. The Hartford Institute has made remarkable progress in improving the nursing care of older adults and in increasing the visibility of geriatric nursing as a specialty area.

There are several people I would like to recognize for the impact they have made on my professional career, as well as on my personal life. Dr. May Futrell, a long-time leader in the field of gerontological nursing, who has recently retired to pursue other dreams, has been a mentor and an inspiration to me for the duration of my entire career as an advanced practice nurse. She has been instrumental in educating many nursing leaders and has had a vision of gerontological nursing as a specialty area at the graduate level since its birth many years ago. Dr. Susan Black, who spent the duration of her career providing quality care to her older adult patients, has been an advocate for the need for health care for all populations. Her enthusiasm for providing quality care for underserved populations has been an inspiration for me. I wish her the best in her new adventures. They have each been instrumental in fostering the education and professional development of many, and we can all be thankful for the years of contribution they have made to older adult health care.

I also feel the importance of recognizing Dr. John Eleftherio, who during his short life provided vision care to so many individuals of all ages. He was especially sensitive to the needs of those with declining vision. He was not aware of the impact he made on my professional career. His support and concern fostered my interest in vision problems.

I also would like to thank my colleagues and friends at the University of Massachusetts Lowell for their support during the editing of this book, which has helped to make it a reality. I am indeed fortunate to work with such a wonderful, talented group of professional nurses.

I would like to thank and express my appreciation to Ramraj Gautam, who has read and helped with the editing of chapters. I appreciate his vision for and enthusiasm about improving the conditions for older adults in all countries and look forward to his leadership in the field of aging in future years.

I would also like to recognize the importance of my family. Thelma and Everett Crocker guided me in the pursuit of excellence and were instrumental in providing me with the strong foundation on which my life and career are built. My brother, Alan, who helps me to maintain a sense of humor, also deserves mention. My husband, Chuck, and my daughters, Courtney and Katelyn, have also provided me with a cornerstone of support, without which I would not be able to pursue my scholarly work. They have endured my long hours at the computer and distraction from their daily life, and accepted this without question. I am thankful to them for encouraging me to pursue those things that are important to me and for providing me with a presence that helps me to balance my professional and personal lives.

Susan Crocker Houde
Editor

VISION LOSS IN OLDER ADULTS

CHAPTER 1

Vision Loss in the Older Adult

An Introduction

Susan Crocker Houde

Vision loss in older adults is a common problem that has a major impact on the social, psychological, and physical functioning of older individuals and their families. Currently, in the United States, 7.3 million adults over 65 years of age report some vision impairment (Arlene R. Gordon Research Institute of Lighthouse International, 2002). The prevalence increases with age with 17% of Americans age 65 and older reporting vision impairment and 26% of Americans 75 years of age and older reporting some problems with vision. The prevalence of vision impairment in the nursing home population has been found to be higher. Twenty-seven percent of nursing home residents 65 years of age and older in the 1997 National Nursing Home Survey were reported to have vision impairment (Gabrel, 2000). An explanation for the higher rate of vision impairment among nursing home residents may be due to the negative effect vision loss has on functional ability, necessitating nursing home placement (Friedman et al., 2004).

As the population in the United States ages, the prevalence of vision impairment is expected to increase. By the year 2010, vision impairment is expected to affect 8.3 million older adults. By 2020, this number is projected to increase to 11.3 million, and by 2030, 14.8 million older adults are expected to be visually impaired (Arlene R. Gordon Research Institute of Lighthouse International, 2002). The expected increased prevalence of vision impairment is related to the predicted increase in the population over the age of 75 to 12% by 2050, from 6% in 2000 (National Center for Health Statistics, 2004).

Vision impairment has been defined as having "20/40 or worse vision in the better eye even with eyeglasses" (Prevent Blindness America, 2002, p. 4) or by self-report from the older adult of:

- the inability to recognize a friend across the room, even when wearing glasses or contact lenses; OR
- inability to read regular newspaper print, even when wearing glasses or contact lenses; OR
- self-rated vision as poor or very poor even when wearing glasses or contact lenses; OR
- report of some other trouble seeing, even when wearing glasses or contact lenses; OR
- blindness in one or both eyes (Arlene R. Gordon Research Institute of Lighthouse International, 2002, p. 2).

The majority of older adults reporting vision impairment are not legally blind. Legal blindness is defined as a "clinically measured visual acuity with best correction in the better eye worse than or equal to 20/200 or a visual field of less than 20 degrees in diameter" (Prevent Blindness America, 2002, p. 4). Of those reporting vision impairment, 11% of those 65 years and older or 3.8 million older adults report severe vision impairment, however (Arlene R. Gordon Research Institute of Lighthouse International, 2002). In the future, because of the aging of the baby boom generation, the number of older adults with severe vision impairment is expected to increase. By the year 2010, the number is projected to reach 4.3 million; by 2020, 5.9 million; and by 2030, it is estimated that 7.7 million older adults will be severely visually impaired in the United States alone (Arlene R. Gordon Research Institute of Lighthouse International).

Severe vision impairment is defined by self-report of:

- inability to recognize a friend at arm's length even when wearing glasses or contact lenses; OR
- inability to read ordinary newspaper print even when wearing glasses or contact lenses, OR
- self-rated vision as poor or very poor even when wearing glasses or contact lenses; OR
- blindness in both eyes (Arlene R. Gordon Research Institute of Lighthouse International, 2002, p. 3).

Globally, vision loss is also a major problem, with 40 million individuals with blindness and 120 million estimated to be visually impaired worldwide

(Sommer, 2004). Many of these individuals are poor with a lack of access to health services. The lack of cataract surgeons in developing countries contributes to approximately 50% of the blindness because of poor access to cataract surgery (Sommer). Nursing involvement in education, advocacy, and policy development has the potential to make a positive impact worldwide on eye health, which can result in a significant positive impact on the quality of life of older adults with chronic eye conditions in all countries, especially those developing countries that presently lack access to adequate eye health care.

IMPACT OF VISION LOSS

There are a number of changes in vision that occur with age that result because of changes in the structure and functioning of the eye. These changes, coupled with eye conditions that have a negative effect on vision, can result in vision loss/impairment that can have adverse social and psychological effects on older adults. The four major causes of vision loss in older adults include age-related macular degeneration, cataracts, glaucoma, and diabetic retinopathy.

Vision loss has been estimated to contribute to difficulty with functioning for 5 million older adults in the United States, and the majority of these individuals reside in the community (AARP, 1997). The limitations that may result because of vision loss may affect the quality of life in an older person by limiting socialization, independence, and the ability to participate in self-care activities (Campbell, Crews, Moriarty, Zack, & Blackman, 1999). Vision loss may also result in changes in family and social roles that may cause stress for the older adult with vision loss and his/her family. Visually impaired older adults have reported greater life problems, increased stress, and a lower level of life satisfaction than those older adults with normal vision (Davies, Lovie-Kitchin, & Thompson, 1995; Horowitz, Reinhardt, Brennan, & Cantor, 1997). Those who report close social friendships have better adaptation to vision loss, better life satisfaction, and less depression than those who do not have close friendship ties, however (Reinhardt, 1996).

There are serious financial implications to society, the family, and the older adult with vision loss. It has been estimated that the direct and indirect costs of the four major causes of vision loss in the older adult are between $30 billion and $40 billion each year (Butler, Faye, Guazzo, & Kupfer, 1997). Despite the high prevalence and high cost of vision loss, reimbursement for visual rehabilitation is usually limited. The cost to the federal government alone for vision impairment and blindness is estimated to be more than $4 billion per year in taxable income and benefits (Prevent Blindness America, 2002).

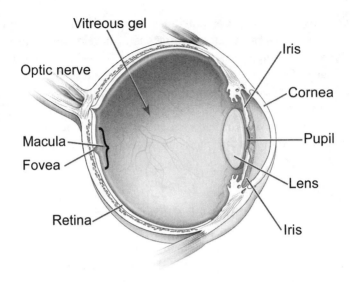

FIGURE 1.1 The eye.
Source: National Eye Institute, National Institutes of Health.

OCULAR AND VISUAL CHANGES WITH AGING

There are a number of structural and physiological changes associated with aging that may result in vision changes affecting functioning of older adults. In fact, all older adults do experience a decrease in their visual ability as they age (Ebersole, Hess, & Luggen, 2004). There are changes that occur in the lens, the retina, the pupil, and the cornea that together have an impact on vision (Figure 1.1). The older adult adapts to many of these changes, and because of their gradual nature he/she may not be aware of the changes in the eye that occur with age. In this section, the changes in the eye that are considered to be normal age-related changes are discussed.

With age, the pupil decreases in size and becomes more fixed. In earlier years, the size of the pupil changes easily in relation to the amount of light in the immediate environment. When levels of light are high, the pupil decreases in size, and when lighting levels are low, the pupil dilates, allowing greater levels of light to reach the retina. Because the maximum size of the pupil decreases with age, the pupil cannot dilate to the same degree as in younger years, resulting in more difficulty in seeing clearly in low light situations for many older adults. This results in requiring higher levels of lighting than younger people. This has important implications for functioning in the home situation, where older adults may need three times more lighting than younger people to function well (Hooyman & Kiyak, 2005). The difficulty older adults experience with light and dark adaptation may predispose them to falls and injury, as they ambulate from room to room with varying light levels and when participating in social activities in the community during the nighttime hours. Difficulty reading signs at night due to low lighting may also be a problem.

Poor tolerance of glare is also a problem for many older adults as they age. Glare from shiny objects in the home, including polished floors, may create a problem for some (Meisami, Brown, & Emerle, 2003). Glare in the home from sunlight may be reduced with curtains and rugs on the floors. Fluorescent lighting may increase glare and may better be replaced with soft lighting with incandescent bulbs (Cleary, 1997).

Difficulty is also often reported with glare from headlights and wet pavement that can make driving at night problematic for older drivers. Frequently night driving is discontinued because of the difficulty with glare, as well as the difficulty with adjustment from dark to light that occurs as one ages (Cleary, 1997). Avoidance of night driving may in turn affect involvement in social activities that occur in the evening.

The cornea of the eye is also affected by aging in that the surface becomes flatter, thicker, and less smooth. This affects the manner in which the light is reflected and may contribute to an increased risk of astigmatism (Ebersole, Hess, & Luggen, 2004). Infection and injury may also be less noticeable in older adults because of a decrease in corneal sensitivity. A diminished corneal reflex may be noted which may have no clinical significance in older adults (Cleary, 1997). It is not uncommon for older adults to develop an arcus senilis, which is a grayish white ring visible on the cornea 1 to 2 mm inside the outer aspect of the iris. It is the accumulation of cholesterol and calcium salts and has no effect on vision. Commonly the iris loses pigmentation with age so that many older adults have grayish or pale blue irises.

The collagen content of the lens in the eye also changes as one ages. Collagen is a protein in the lens that becomes thicker and harder with age. New cells continue to be produced in the lens capsule as one ages and the accumulation of old cells in the lens capsule along with the new cells contributes to lens thickening. This process results in a decrease in the elasticity of the lens that causes a decrease in the ability of the lens to change its shape. The functional ability of the ciliary muscles that work to change the shape of the lens also decreases. The muscles shorten due to atrophy and connective tissue replaces the lost muscle. These changes in the lens and ciliary muscles result in a decline in the eye's accommodation capacity. Accommodation is the process whereby one adjusts focus from near objects to far objects and back to near objects easily. Commonly one begins to experience difficulty in the ability to accommodate by the time they reach the age of 40 or 50, and it continues to progress into and throughout old age. This condition, known as presbyopia, results in the need to hold reading materials further away in order to focus clearly on the print. Glasses can help one focus for reading purposes, but difficulty may result when there is a need for changing focus rapidly, such as when one is looking at notes and glancing at an audience, or writing notes and glancing at a speaker. This difficulty occurs because glasses may help one focus on close objects, but do not assist in the problem one experiences when there is a need to change focal points.

Not only is accommodation affected by aging changes in the lens, but also the lens thickening resulting from an increase in the lens density contributes to visual changes. This increased lens thickness decreases the size of the anterior chamber of the eye that may result in a loss of the efficiency by which the resorption of intraocular fluid occurs, resulting in the potential for an increase in intraocular pressure. The aging changes in the lens also contribute to a decrease in the transparency of the lens. Generally the aging changes in the lens do not occur uniformly and result in an uneven passage of light onto the retina, which in turn contributes to glare sensitivity as previously discussed. The uneven passage of light onto the retina may also contribute to difficulty in depth perception that may result in difficulty with driving, especially during nighttime hours. The lens changes become severe in some individuals so that there is clouding of the lens that prohibits light from entering the eye, in a condition known as cataracts.

The loss of transparency in the lens may contribute to a decrease in the ability to discriminate colors, especially shades of blue and green, as well as a need for lenses for reading. Changes in the transparency of the lens may result because of a yellowing of the lens, compression of the lens fibers, and poor nutrition to the lens because of a decrease in the efficiency of the aqueous humor. Changes in the retina may also contribute to difficulty in distinguishing darker colors such as blues, purples, and greens. Color clarity decreases in over half of the older adult population by the time they are in their 80s (Ebersole et al., 2004).

Some older adults experience a decrease in the secretion of tears with a sense of dry eyes. Eye lubrication also decreases because the number of goblet cells in the conjunctiva that are responsible for mucin, which assists with eye lubrication, diminishes. This condition may be annoying for older adults in that the eyes may feel irritated, but is not a serious condition and can be relieved with the application of artificial tears that can be purchased over the counter. There may also be a drooping of the eyelids due to the loss of elasticity and atrophy of the skin that may interfere with vision, if it is severe enough. A loss of strength in the orbital muscles may also result in the eyelids turning inward or outward. An ectropian may contribute to dryness of the eyes because there is an eversion of the lower lid that may result in poor closure of the eye with sleep. An entropian, on the other hand, occurs when spasms of the orbicular muscle result in the lower lid turning inward, resulting in irritation of the eyeball by the lower eyelashes.

Not only does the functioning of the ciliary muscles deteriorate, but also the elevator muscle functioning also declines. This decline results in a decreased ability to look upward and may affect one's ability to read overhead signs or see objects that are above eye level. This may contribute to a narrowing of the visual field that occurs with aging, in that the peripheral vision of older adults is not as wide as that in younger age groups. This may be a very subtle change and may not be detected. For others, the loss of peripheral vision may result in a limitation in social and physical activities, as well as a problem driving, because of difficulties seeing other cars not visible in the decreased visual field. The depth of the anterior chamber changes with age because of a thickening of the lens. This coupled with a decreased efficiency in resorbing intraocular fluid may contribute to a higher risk of developing glaucoma as one ages, which results in more marked changes in peripheral vision over time if not adequately treated.

Another occurrence that may be an annoyance to older adults is the development of vitreous floaters, which are opacities visible in one's visual field that appear as specks, webs, or lines that move with eye movement. These floaters occur as the vitreous loses water with aging, and are the result of vitreous that has separated from the retina. The annoyance that one experiences from floaters generally diminishes with time and does not affect visual acuity. However, the rapid onset of multiple floaters sometimes accompanied by a flash of light may indicate a detached retina and should be promptly evaluated.

CAUSES OF AGE-RELATED VISION LOSS

Age-Related Macular Degeneration

Age-related macular degeneration (AMD) is the leading cause of irreversible vision loss and blindness in older Americans (Prevent Blindness America, 2002). In fact, based on population estimates from the 2000 census, approximately 1.7 million persons in the United States that are age 65 and older have some vision impairment that is the result of AMD (Arlene R. Gordon Research Institute of Lighthouse International, 2002). Decreases in vision because of age-related macular degeneration are expected to increase in the future (American

Foundation for the Blind, 1999). From data collected in an Australian study, it was estimated that one in three persons 70 years of age and older would have lesions typical of AMD over 5 years and that there would be progression to a more severe form of the condition after the age of 80 (Mukesh et al., 2004). Because of the high incidence of AMD in this study, the authors called for the need for preventive strategies to reduce the vision impairment that often results from this condition.

With AMD there may be a loss of central vision caused by atrophy, scarring, and hemorrhages in the macula. Not all older adults with AMD experience severe vision loss. There are two types of AMD: nonexudative or dry AMD and exudative or wet AMD. The nonexudative type of AMD is less likely to progress to severe impairment and is characterized by yellow deposits of extracellular material in the macula that are known as drusen, which are usually asymptomatic. Areas of retinal atrophy that appear as oval or round patches may lead to vision loss over time. Nonexudative AMD is the most common type of AMD. The exudative type of AMD is more rapidly progressive and results in the proliferation of abnormal blood vessels that leak blood and fluid into the macula, resulting in central vision loss. Central vision loss can have negative psychological and social effects on older adults because of the loss of functional ability and the need for older adults to adapt their activities because of the inability to see detail closely.

Based on the 2000 U.S. Census, it has been estimated that 960,000 individuals have advanced AMD in one eye. Furthermore, it was predicted that 1,315,000 of those age 55 and older in the United States would develop AMD within 5 years and that 8,045,000 were at high risk of developing AMD (Age-Related Eye Disease Study Research Group, 2003). Because there is presently no known cure for AMD, the need to prevent this serious eye condition is of paramount importance. These projections have clear implications for the importance of the role of the nurse in educating the public about what is known about the problem and strategies to help prevent the occurrence and progression of this disorder, which can adversely affect quality of life in the older adult. Data regarding the role of antioxidants in the prevention of AMD are accumulating, and knowledge about current research should be incorporated into nursing practice.

Cataracts

Both in the United States and worldwide, cataracts are a common cause of vision loss and blindness. In the United States, cataracts occur in more than 50% of adults by the age of 80 and are more common in females than males (Prevent Blindness America, 2002). The most frequently performed surgery for

Medicare beneficiaries in the United States is cataract surgery, and 43% of the office visits to ophthalmologists and optometrists for Medicare beneficiaries are for older adults with cataracts (National Advisory Eye Council, 1998). The World Health Organization (2004a) estimates that cataracts result in blindness for 16 million individuals worldwide every year, and is the leading cause of blindness in the world. In a study that described the incidence of visual impairment in an Afro-Caribbean population, it was found that the incidence of visual impairment was high among this population of older adults and that cataracts was the cause of 52% of the blindness alone, and another 10% of those blind had both cataracts and glaucoma (Leske et al., 2004). In a nursing home population in the United States, African American residents, compared to White residents, have been found to have a higher incidence of unoperated cataracts, but the incidence of cataracts was high among all nursing home residents (Friedman et al., 2004). There has been difficulty noted in reporting the true prevalence of cataract in older adults because many do not have vision impairment from the cataract that is severe enough to warrant surgery (Arlene R. Gordon Research Institute of Lighthouse International, 2002; National Advisory Eye Council, 1993).

Cataracts occur as the lens of the eye becomes cloudy and yellowish with aging. Normally the lens is clear, but because of protein aggregation in the lens capsule there is a loss of transparency (Kalina, 1997). This change results in blurring of vision and glare that is usually slowly progressive. In the United States, the Medicare program spends more than $3.4 billion treating cataracts each year (Prevent Blindness America, 2002).

Glaucoma

Glaucoma is considered to be the second leading cause of blindness worldwide (Standefer, 2004), being responsible for over 5 million cases of blindness (World Health Organization, 2004b). It is estimated that 1% to 2% of the world population has chronic glaucoma (World Health Organization, 2004c). In the United States, approximately 3 million individuals have glaucoma, many of whom are older adults (Glaucoma Research Foundation, 2006). It is more common in Blacks (Prevent Blindness America, 2002) and has been found to be a leading cause of blindness in Hispanics (Rodriquez, 2002).

Glaucoma is the result of damage to the optic disc and nerve because of increased intraocular pressure. The increase in pressure is caused by an obstruction of the outflow of aqueous humor through the anterior chamber angle. There are two types of glaucoma: primary open-angle glaucoma and primary angle-closure glaucoma. Primary open-angle glaucoma is by far the most common type seen in older adults and accounts for at least 90% of the cases (Kalina, 1997). Changes that occur in primary open-angle glaucoma are the result of increased intraocular pressure and are chronic, asymptomatic, and slowly progressive (Quillen, 1999). The increase in intraocular pressure may cause permanent loss of peripheral vision before the individual notes a change in vision. Primary angle-closure glaucoma occurs in less than 10% of cases, and is more common in Asian populations (Kalina). It is an acute condition that results in a sudden blockage of the outflow of aqueous from the anterior chamber as a result of thickening of the iris. Symptoms are se- vere and sudden and include pain in the eye area, blurry vision, and seeing halos around lights. Primary angle-closure glaucoma is a medical emergency. Screening for glaucoma is very important, as early detection and treatment can prevent the vision loss that is commonly the result, if the condition is left untreated.

Diabetic Retinopathy

Diabetes mellitus is a common health problem in the United States. It is esti- mated that there are 18.2 million individuals who have the disease in the United States (American Diabetes Association, 2005), of whom 5.3 million have dia- betic retinopathy (Prevent Blindness America, 2002). Diabetic retinopathy is the leading cause of legal blindness in adults younger than the age of 75, and is more common in African Americans (American Diabetes Association) and Hispanics (Prevent Blindness America). The incidence of diabetic retinopathy typically increases with the length of time one has diabetes mellitus (Kalina, 1997; Quillen, 1999). The degree and rate of progression of the retinopa- thy correlate strongly with the level and duration of the elevated blood sugar (Winters & Jernigan, 2000). Good control of blood sugars in individuals with diabetes mellitus has been shown to decrease the incidence and delay the progression of diabetic retinopathy (Diabetes Control and Complications Trial Research Group, 1993).

Diabetic retinopathy may be either nonproliferative or proliferative. In nonproliferative diabetic retinopathy, abnormalities in the retinal circulation are evident that may include cotton wool spots, microaneurysms, hemorrhages, retinal edema, exudates, and other microvascular abnormalities. Proliferative retinopathy results from a progression of nonproliferative retinopathy and is characterized by the proliferation of new blood vessels and fibrous tissue on the retina. It may remain asymptomatic until the traction of vessels on the retina results in a vitreous hemorrhage (Elner, 1999). The nurse's role in early detection and effective treatment of diabetes mellitus can have a major impact on the prevention of vision loss from diabetic retinopathy.

THE ROLE OF THE PROFESSIONAL NURSE—AN OVERVIEW

The nurse's role in the care of older adults with vision problems is multi-faceted and includes education, advocacy, support, assessment, and research (Houde & Huff, 2003; Houde, 2001). The educational role is an important one. Educating older adults with vision problems and their families about the diagnosis, treatment, resources, and assistive devices may help the older individual cope with the changes that occur as a result of visual problems. Strategies to prevent or delay the progression of the disorder may also be an important educational priority. The need for preventive care and screening may also be instrumental in avoiding vision loss in the older adult population.

Advocacy, both on behalf of older adults with vision loss and motivating older adults to become their own advocate, is also an important role of the nurse. Educating legislators about the needs of older adults with vision loss may go a long way in assisting legislators to make informed decisions about funding and programs that may assist those with vision loss and their families. Motivating older adults to prepare for anticipated vision loss and to seek needed services are also important roles that can promote the sense of empowerment over the challenge of age-related vision loss.

Providing emotional support and helping older adults mobilize a support network can be instrumental in preventing loneliness and promoting adaptation to vision loss for those residing in the community. Assessment for changes in vision, mobility or functional problems, social or service needs, and adjustment disorders or depression are essential for providing comprehensive care for the older adult, and his or her family, with age-related vision problems.

There is a need for professional nurses to become involved in research related to the care of older adults with vision loss. Evaluation of programs and interventions to support those with vision loss will be needed to determine the optimal strategies for promoting quality of life in this population. Data that support the effectiveness of specific programs are essential to increase funding for services to those who are visually impaired. Involvement in intervention studies by nurses knowledgeable about age-related vision loss and the impact it has on older adults and their families can greatly increase the clinical and policy relevance of study results.

REFERENCES

AARP, Program Resources Dept. and Administration on Aging. (1997). *Profile of older Americans*. Washington, DC: U.S. Department of Health and Human Services.

Age-Related Eye Disease Study Research Group. (2003). Potential public health impact of Age-Related Eye Disease Study results: AREDS Report No. 11. *Archives of Ophthalmology, 121*(11), 1621–1624.

American Diabetes Association. (2005). *All about diabetes*. Retrieved January 22, 2005, from http://www.diabetes.org/about-diabetes.jsp

American Foundation for the Blind. (1999). *USABLE data report: Using statistics about blindness and low vision effectively*. Retrieved October 31, 1999, from http://www.afb.org/j_usable1999.html

Arlene R. Gordon Research Institute of Lighthouse International. (2002). *Statistics on vision impairment: A resource manual*. Retrieved May 13, 2006, from http://ww.lighthouse.org/downloads/researchstats.rtf

Butler, R., Faye, E., Guazzo, E., & Kupfer, C. (1997). Keeping an eye on vision: Primary care of age-related ocular disease. *Geriatrics, 52*(8), 30–38.

Campbell, V. A., Crews, J. E., Moriarty, D. G., Zack, M. M., & Blackman, D. K. (1999). *Surveillance for sensory impairment, activity limitation, and health related quality of life among older adults — United States, 1993–1997*. MMWR Surveillance Summaries, December 17, 1999/48 (SS08), 131–156. Retrieved February 13, 2003, from http://www.cdc.gov/epo/mmwr/preview/mmwrhtml/SS4808a6.htm

Cleary, B. (1997). Age-related changes on the special senses. In M. A. Matteson, E. S. McConnell, & A. D. Linton (Eds.), *Gerontological nursing: Concepts and practice* (pp. 385–405). Philadelphia, PA: Saunders.

Davies, C., Lovie-Kitchin, J., & Thompson, B. (1995). Psychosocial adjustment to age-related macular degeneration. *Journal of Visual Impairment and Blindness, 89*(1), 16–27.

Diabetes Control and Complications Trial Research Group. (1993). The effect of intensive treatment of diabetes in the development and progression of long-term complications in insulin-dependent diabetes mellitus. *New England Journal of Medicine, 329*, 977–986.

Ebersole, P., Hess, P., & Luggen, A. (2004). *Toward healthy aging: Human needs and nursing response*. St. Louis, MO: Mosby.

Elner, S. (1999). Gradual painless vision loss: Retinal causes. *Clinics in Geriatric Medicine, 15*(1), 25–46.

Friedman, D., West, S., Munoz, B., Park, W., Deremeik, J., Massof, R., et al. (2004). Racial variations in causes of vision loss in nursing homes: The Salisbury Eye Evaluation in Nursing Home Groups (SEEING) Study. *Archives of Ophthalmology, 122*(7), 1019–1024.

Gabrel, S. (2000). Characteristics of elderly nursing home current residents and discharges: Data from the 1997 National Nursing Home Survey. *Advance Data*. (No. 312).

Glaucoma Research Foundation. (2006). *Glaucoma facts and stats*. Retrieved May 13, 2006, from http://www.glaucoma.org/learn/glaucoma_facts.html.

Hooyman, N., & Kiyak, A. A. (2005). *Social gerontology: A multidisciplinary perspective*. Boston: Allyn & Bacon.

Horowitz, A., Reinhardt, J. P., Brennan, M., & Cantor, M. (1997). *Aging and vision loss: Experiences, attitudes, and knowledge of older Americans.* New York: Arlene R. Gordon Research Institute, The Lighthouse, Inc.

Houde, S. (2001). Age-related vision loss in the older adult: The role of the nurse practitioner in prevention and early detection. *Clinical Excellence for Nurse Practitioners, 5*(4), 185–195.

Houde, S., & Huff, M. (2003). Age-related vision loss in older adults: A challenge for gerontological nurses. *Journal of Gerontological Nursing, 29*(4), 25–33.

Kalina, R. (1997). Seeing into the future: Vision and aging. *Western Journal of Medicine, 167*(4), 253–257.

Leske, M., Wu, S., Hyman, L., Nemesure, B., Hennis, A., Schachat, A., et al. (2004). Four-year incidence of visual impairment: Barbados Incidence Study of Eye Diseases. *Ophthalmology, 111*(1), 118–124.

Meisami, E., Brown, C. M., & Emerle, H. F. (2003). Sensory systems: Normal aging disorders, and treatments of vision and hearing in humans. In P. S. Timoras (Ed.), *Physiological basis of aging and geriatrics* (pp. 141–165). Boca Raton, FL: CRC Press.

Mukesh, B., Dimitrov, P., Leikin, S., Wang, J., Mitchell, P., McCarty, C., et al. (2004). Five-year incidence of age-related maculopathy: The Visual Impairment Project. *Ophthalmology, 111*(6), 1176–1182.

National Advisory Eye Council. (1993). *Vision research—A national plan: 1994–1998.* (NIH Publication No. 95-3186). Bethesda, MD: National Institutes of Health.

National Advisory Eye Council. (1998). *Vision research—A national plan: 1999–2003.* (NIH Publication No. 98-4120). Bethesda, MD: National Institutes of Health.

National Center for Health Statistics. (2004). *Health, United States, 2004.* Hyattsville, MD: National Center fir Health Statistics. Retrieved January 22, 2005, from http://www.cdc.gov/nchs/data/hus/hus0trend.pdf#exe.

Prevent Blindness America. (2002). *Vision problems in the U.S.* Schaumburg, IL: Prevent Blindness America. Retrieved July 28, 2004, from http://www.preventblindness.org/vpus/vp.html.

Quillen, D. (1999). Common causes of vision loss in elderly patients. *American Family Physician, 60*(1), 99–108.

Reinhardt, J. (1996). The importance of friendship and family support in adaptation to chronic vision impairment. *Journal of Gerontology: Social Sciences, 51B*(5), P268–P278.

Rodriquez, J. (2002). Causes of blindness and visual impairment in a population-based sample of U.S. Hispanics. *Ophthalmology, 109,* 737–743.

Sommer, A. (2004). Global health, global vision. *Archives of Ophthalmology, 122*(6), 911–912.

Standefer, J. E. (2004). Glaucoma is second leading cause if blindness globally. *In Focus, 82,* 887–888. Retrieved February 15, 2005, from www.who.int/bulletin/bulletin-board/83/infocus11041/en.

Winters, S., & Jernigan, V. (2000). Vascular disease risk markers in diabetes: Monitoring and intervention. *The Nurse Practitioner, 25*(6), 40, 43–44, 46.

World Health Organization. (2004a). *Cataracts.* Retrieved September 14, 2004, from http://www.who.int/uv/faq/uvhealthfac/en/index3.htm.

World Health Organization. (2004b). *Guidelines for disease control.* Retrieved February 15, 2005, from http://www.who.int/pbd/publications/guidelines/en/.

World Health Organization. (2004c). *Bulletin of World Health Organization,* 82, 811–890. Retrieved February 15, 2005, from http://www.who.int/bulletin/volumes/82/11/feature1104/en/index1.html.

CHAPTER 2

Age-Related Macular Degeneration

Ruth Remington

It is a well-known fact that the number of persons over the age of 60 is increasing at a startling rate. People over age 60 constitute an estimated 20% of the population in the developed regions of the world. Consequently, chronic illness has emerged as a major cause of disability and activity restriction in the aging population. Age-related macular degeneration (AMD) is the leading cause of vision-related disability in the Western world, affecting between 1.8 million and 14 million people in the United States (Congdon, Friedman, & Lietman, 2003; Moshfeghi & Lewis, 2003; Tasman & Rovner, 2004) and 20 million to 25 million people worldwide (Chopdar, Chakravarthy, & Verma, 2003). It is the cause of partial vision loss for 1 of every 28 U.S. residents and is more prevalent among Whites and Hispanics than Blacks (The Eye Diseases Prevalence Research Group, 2004).

Visual deficits increase considerably with age for persons of all races and ethnicities. Persons 80 or more years of age comprise approximately 8% of the population, yet represent nearly 70% of all blindness (The Eye Diseases Prevalence Research Group, 2004). Among individuals over the age of 75, up to 41% have some limitation in function due to AMD (Seddon, Cote, & Rosner, 2003). Older adults often need to adapt to living with limitations imposed by more than one chronic illness, and the care of these individuals is increasingly entrusted to nurses (Moore, 2001). This chapter presents information about the disease pathophysiology, diagnosis, and medical management of AMD, for the purpose of helping nurses plan quality care to a growing segment of society.

PATHOPHYSIOLOGY

AMD

AMD is a progressive disorder of the macula, which is the light-sensitive area of the retina. The macula, which has no blood supply, is responsible for detailed, focused central vision. This area contains the rods and cones that gather light and convert it to nerve impulses that are transmitted to the brain via the optic nerve. Under the macula, the retinal pigment epithelium (RPE) and its membrane maintain the barrier between the choroid and the retina. The choroid, which lies between the retina and the sclera, is the source of blood supply for the retina (Chopdar, Chakravarthy, & Verma, 2003; Moore, 2001; Moshfeghi & Lewis, 2003).

As people age, the RPE become less efficient in supplying nourishment to the retinal cells and removing waste products. The cells of the RPE gradually degenerate and atrophy, causing a painless loss of central vision. As metabolic waste products accumulate, yellow fatty deposits, called drusen, build up in the retina. Drusen do not affect vision, and not all people with drusen develop AMD. However, drusen must be present for AMD to develop (Chopdar et al., 2003; Moshfeghi & Lewis, 2003; Sadler, 2002). There are two types of AMD: atrophic or "dry" type and exudative or "wet" type. The dry type is the most common, accounting for 80% to 85% of cases, but the wet type accounts for 90% of severe vision loss from the disease (Moshfeghi & Lewis).

Dry AMD

Over time, drusen deposits enlarge, causing the RPE and photoreceptors to deteriorate due to a lack of nutrients. This results in a gradual loss of central visual acuity. Vision loss from dry AMD progresses slowly over 5 to 10 years, sometimes causing severe vision loss, but rarely results in total blindness. This form of the disease often develops in both eyes, and over time can develop into wet AMD (Chopdar et al., 2003; Moore, 2001; Moshfeghi & Lewis, 2003). To date there is no treatment that will cure or improve vision of individuals with the dry form of AMD.

Wet AMD

Exudative or wet, AMD is characterized by the formation of abnormal blood vessels (neovascularization) under the retina in the choroid. These blood vessels may bleed and leak fluid, blood, or lipids into the macula, causing blurred, distorted central vision. Scar tissue forms causing permanent blind spots in the center of the visual field. This form of AMD can progress rapidly causing sudden, permanent vision loss (Chopdar et al., 2003; Moore, 2001; Moshfeghi & Lewis, 2003).

RISK FACTORS

Despite considerable research, the cause of AMD remains unclear. Epidemiologic studies have proposed many risk factors for AMD, and only a few have been consistently shown to be related to the onset of AMD. These include advanced age, White race, and smoking. The person who has drusen, macular changes, or neovascularization in one eye is at greater risk of developing it in the other eye. Exposure to ultraviolet light, family history, and diet have been suspected, but remain unproven, in the development of AMD.

Age is the strongest nonmodifiable risk factor for AMD. Studies have repeatedly shown a direct relationship between advancing age and increased incidence of AMD. Smoking is the strongest modifiable risk factor for AMD. The effects of smoking and hypertension on the blood vessels of the cardiovascular system are well known. Smoking also damages the blood vessels of the eye (McGrory & Remington, 2004; Moore, 2001). Studies consistently demonstrate a relationship between smoking and the development of AMD. Current and former smokers have a two to threefold greater risk of developing the condition than those who never smoked. The risk associated with past smoking does not decrease for 15 to 20 years after quitting (Delcourt, Diaz, Ponton-Sanchez, & Papoz, 1998; Seddon, Willett, Speizer, & Hankinson, 1996).

The Age-Related Eye Disease Study (AREDS, 2001), a recently completed, multicenter clinical trial, demonstrated that high doses of antioxidants or zinc, alone or in combination, produced a significant reduction in the risk of progression to advanced AMD. The benefit was increased for those who took both supplements simultaneously. No preventive benefit was observed for persons without evidence of the disease.

Studies examining the relationship between sun exposure and increased incidence of AMD have been inconclusive. A protective effect of hat and sunglasses on the development of drusen and depigmentation of the RPE has been suggested (Tomany, Cruickshanks, Klein, Klein, & Knudtson, 2004). Dietary fat intake and family history might be related to the development of AMD; however, results have been inconclusive (Moore, 2001; Rowe, MacLean, & Shekelle, 2004; Seddon, Cote, & Rosner, 2003). Research suggests that statins, used to lower lipid levels, have a protective effect against the development of AMD, but again, results are uncertain (Hall, Gale, Sydall, Phillips, & Marlyn, 2001).

SYMPTOMS

Regardless of the type of AMD, the symptoms are similar. With both wet and dry AMD, central vision is lost and vision becomes distorted. Peripheral vision remains intact. The onset and intensity of visual symptoms differ according to the type of AMD.

Initial visual changes may be so subtle for individuals who have the dry type of AMD that they may not be aware that they have the disease. In the early stage, the person may be aware of slight blurring of vision, needing more light for reading or doing close work. Older adults may not notice early changes in vision or may dismiss the changes as part of the aging process. Dry AMD usually starts in one eye, and over time, develops in the other eye, but may progress at a different rate in each eye. The person may experience difficulty driving, watching television, or performing tasks that call for the ability to see detail. As the disease progresses, damage to the macula causes localized areas of vision loss, called scotoma, appearing in the center of the visual field. Vision becomes distorted, as straight lines appear wavy (metamorphosia). These changes can significantly interfere with the ability to recognize people, read, and perform activities of daily living. Color vision and depth perception may deteriorate, making objects appear washed out or disappear from view. Individuals retain their peripheral vision, which can allow them to continue to perform many daily tasks (Chopdar et al., 2003; Miller, 2004; Moore, 2001; Moshefeghi & Lewis, 2003).

The neovascularization of wet AMD can occur without symptoms in some people. If the new blood vessels leak blood and fluid into the macula, causing it to bulge, the central vision may become distorted. With hemorrhage, visual changes can include a haze obscuring vision, floaters, and flashing lights. Those who have the wet type of AMD can experience a sudden onset of symptoms. Wet AMD can progress rapidly and cause permanent visual loss. The older adult may report a sudden distortion of central vision, and progress over several weeks or months until a scar is formed preventing further loss. Often, legal blindness has occurred in the affected eye by the time scarring is completed. Even in the absence of symptoms, once the exudative changes of wet AMD have developed, the individual is at high risk for the same changes in the other eye, making regular eye exams essential (Arnold & Sarks, 2000; Chopdar et al., 2003; McGrory & Remington, 2004; Moshfeghi & Lewis, 2003).

DIAGNOSIS

A comprehensive evaluation for AMD begins with a focused history. The nurse working with older adults should assess for risk factors of AMD including family history and smoking history. Subtle vision changes in the older adult should not be dismissed as part of the normal aging process. Family members' input can be helpful to supplement the patient's data regarding symptoms of vision loss. In addition to medication history, vitamin and over-the-counter medication use should be evaluated, as many times these supplements are not considered drugs by the older adult. Some of the over-the-counter medications taken frequently by older adults can cause visual changes. Antihistamines (Benadryl, Allegra) can lead to dry eyes and decreased vision. Anti-inflammatory medications, such as Advil and Aleve, can cause decreased or blurred vision (Miller, 2004).

Early detection of AMD is essential to maintain ocular health. Although currently available therapies do not cure the disease, the progression can be slowed, and efforts to preserve vision are crucial (Moore, 2001). Diagnostic evaluation should begin with assessment of visual acuity for near and far vision. Color perception can be easily evaluated using the Ishihara color plates. This is the most common screening test for color vision anomalies. The Ishihara color plates are a series of images on which letters or numbers are printed in dots of primary colors, surrounded by dots of secondary colors (Pache et al., 2003). Older adults with normal vision are able to distinguish the letter or number imbedded in the image, whereas those with AMD have more difficulty identifying colors because color identification occurs in the central vision (Smeltzer & Bare, 2004).

To detect metamorphosia in AMD, older adults should be asked to view an Amsler grid (Figure 2.1). This is a screening test for AMD that is made up of a series of vertical and horizontal lines that form a grid pattern. The older adult is asked to cover one eye and focus on a dot in the center of the grid. Corrective lenses are worn during the exam. If the vertical or horizontal lines do not appear to be straight and wavy lines are perceived, or a dark spot in the center of the grid is seen, the presence of AMD is a concern. Individuals with AMD should be given the Amsler grid to take home and use daily to identify visual changes early. Any changes when viewing the Amsler grid should be reported to the health care provider immediately. The internal structures of the eye should be evaluated by ophthalmoscopic examination. Older adults should be referred to an ophthalmologist for a dilated examination at least yearly. Drusen, choriodal neovascularization, leaking blood and fluid, and scarring may be identified. On fundoscopic exam, drusen appear as small yellow deposits with distinct edges in the fundus, most commonly in the

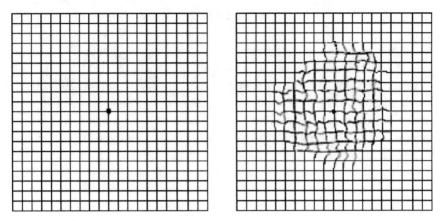

FIGURE 2.1 Amsler grid as seen with normal vision and with age-related macular degeneration.
Source: National Eye Institute, National Institutes of Health.

macula. Over time these drusen can coalesce, leading to atrophy of the macula. Choroidal neovascularization may have several presentations. These new vessels are very narrow and appear in a disorderly fashion on the retina and may extend into the vitreous. Neovascularization also may be seen as a pigment epithelial detachment, or a dome-shaped elevation of the RPE, much like a blister. Hemorrhages may appear like red dots, smudges, or flame shapes. A scar is characterized by atrophy and lipid exudate (Moshfeghi & Lewis, 2003).

Individuals suspected of having wet AMD because of choroidal neovascularization or hemorrhage should undergo angiographic imaging of the retina and choroid by an ophthalmologist. Fluorescein or indocyanine dye is injected intravenously, usually in a vein in the antecubital area. The dye can be seen in the retina within 10 to 15 seconds. A series of photographs is taken of the back of the eye over 10 to 30 minutes, using a specially designed camera. Choroidal neovascularization and leakage can be identified in the photographs. This procedure also allows for precise monitoring of the progression of the disease with repeated photographs over time (Chopdar et al., 2003; Moore, 2001; Moshfeghi & Lewis, 2003). The patient should be instructed that the skin may appear to have a gold tone, and the urine may be deep yellow or orange for 24 hours following the procedure until the dye is excreted (Smeltzer & Bare, 2004).

MEDICAL MANAGEMENT

Currently there is no treatment that is known to prevent or cure AMD. Therapeutic options to control the disease are limited, but research is being conducted on therapeutic modalities that may delay the progression of the condition and may help to maintain the quality of life of those with AMD. With the increase in the older population, we can expect a comparable increase in AMD. Dissemination of strategies to maintain ocular health is essential. Measures such as regular eye examinations for adults over 50 years of age, smoking cessation, blood pressure control, and use of hats and sunglasses when outdoors have been suggested as reasonable strategies that may have a positive effect on preserving vision and promoting general health (Eye Diseases Prevalence Research Group, 2004). Older adults may benefit from teaching about the importance of a low-fat diet as a means of maintaining good eye and cardiovascular health (Seddon et al., 2003). Studies are being conducted by nurses and others in the health care field in the areas of nutrition, nutritional supplements, and other holistic therapies to promote and maintain eye health. To provide holistic nursing care, nurses need to become educated in the advances in nutritional health and supplements (Smeeding, 2001).

Antioxidant and Zinc Supplements

Dietary modification and nutritional supplementation are approaches that show promise for slowing the progression of AMD. Findings of the AREDS (2001), a major clinical trial sponsored by the National Eye Institute, support the promotion of high doses of antioxidant vitamins and zinc in older adults with AMD. These nutrients may not prevent the development of AMD or restore vision lost to the disease in those who are already affected; however, in large enough doses, they may help to slow the progression to advanced AMD. AREDS was a randomized, placebo-controlled, double-masked clinical trial in which 3,640 adults ages 55 to 80 participated in the AMD portion of the study. Participants were assigned to receive one of four treatments: (a) zinc, 80 mg; (b) antioxidants (vitamin C, 500 mg; vitamin E, 400 IU; and beta carotene, 15 mg); (c) antioxidants plus zinc; or (d) placebo. Participants were followed for an average of 6.3 years. Compliance with the assigned treatment was good, estimated at 75%.

Results of the study showed no benefit of the treatment for persons with no AMD or early AMD. For persons with intermediate AMD in one or both eyes, or advanced AMD in one eye, there was a significant decrease in the risk of developing advanced AMD in each of the three experimental treatment groups over the placebo group. The reduction in risk for advanced AMD for those taking antioxidants and zinc was 25%; for those taking zinc alone, 21%; and for those taking antioxidants alone, 17%. The chance of developing vision loss from advanced AMD was 23% in the group who took antioxidants plus zinc and 29% in the placebo group. Overall there were no significant serious adverse effects reported from taking the supplements, although there were more hospitalizations for genitourinary disorders for participants taking zinc (Age-Related Eye Disease Study Research Group, 2001).

Implications of the AREDS are that persons over 55 years old have a dilated eye exam to determine their risk for developing AMD. Those who have intermediate or advanced AMD or vision loss due to AMD should consider taking high-dose antioxidants plus zinc on a daily basis. Doses used in the study were 500 mg of vitamin C, 400 IU of vitamin E, 15 mg of beta carotene (25,000 IU vitamin A), and 80 mg of zinc. Copper, 2 mg, was added to the zinc because high doses of zinc are associated with copper deficiency. Smokers have demonstrated an increased incidence of lung cancer when assigned to beta carotene supplementation in other studies, and it may be reasonable to recommend that smokers avoid beta carotene. Because no benefit was shown for those who do not have AMD, high-dose supplementation is not recommended, and a multivitamin should be sufficient (Age-Related Eye Diseases Study Research Group, 2001).

Recent attention has focused on the potential for lutein and zeaxanthin to slow the development of age-related eye disease. These are plant pigments from the carotenoid family, like beta carotene, that are concentrated in the macula. Unlike beta carotene, they cannot form vitamin A. Their importance to eye tissues may be that they are the only carotenoids in the eye, whereas other body tissues contain a variety of carotenoids. Research is ongoing and inconclusive at this point (Mares, La Rowe, & Blodi, 2004).

Laser Photocoagulation

Laser photocoagulation of abnormal choroidal blood vessels has been shown to reduce the risk of severe vision loss due to AMD in a small number of people with wet AMD. This is the first effective treatment for the exudative form of AMD (Fine, Berger, Maguire, & Ho, 2000). The procedure is painless and usually done on an outpatient basis, taking less than 30 minutes. The pupil is dilated and anesthetized, and a high-energy laser beam is directed at the abnormal blood vessels in the macula for the purpose of sealing them. Laser, however, destroys the surrounding retina, and the resulting scar causes a corresponding defect in the central visual field. This scar causes an immediate and permanent reduction in vision. However, this vision loss is less than that which would eventually occur if the eye had been left untreated (Arnold & Sarks, 2000; Chopdar et al., 2003; Moshfeghi & Lewis, 2003). The procedure is effective in only 10% to 15% of cases, and there is a 50% chance of recurrence within 2 years (Fine et al.). The patient will need to wear sunglasses following the procedure, as the pupil will remain dilated for several hours.

Photodynamic Therapy

Laser therapy is only effective in the avascular area of the fovea. Because most neovascularization extends outside the fovea, a procedure has been developed in which a photosensitizing drug, verteporfin (Visudyne), is activated by laser. In two randomized, placebo-controlled trials, patients treated with verteporfin prior to laser therapy had less visual loss than those who received a placebo. The benefit persisted 2 years after the treatment (Fine et al., 2000). Photodynamic therapy (PDT) can reduce the risk of vision loss due to wet AMD by 30% to 50% (Ferris, 2004).

Verteporfin is injected intravenously in the arm over 10 minutes. The dye pools in the damaged vessels of the choroid. Five minutes after the injection, the eye is anesthetized. At 15 minutes, the dye is activated by a laser, sealing off the leaky vessels. Because the dye does not get into the healthy tissue or the retinal cells, these cells do not react to the laser, preserving retinal tissue. The patient can go home in about 4 to 5 hours. The treatment is repeated in 3 months, and over a 2-year period, individuals generally receive five to six treatments (Moshfeghi & Lewis, 2003; Watkins, 2005).

After the treatment, the dye remains in the body for 24 hours. The older adult will be photosensitive for about 5 days. Because the dye was injected into the systemic circulation, it can reach the capillaries of the skin and become activated by sunlight. The nurse should instruct the patient to wear sunglasses, a hat, long-sleeved shirt, and slacks for 5 days. Also, the patient should be instructed to avoid direct sunlight for 5 days to prevent potentially severe blistering sunburn. The person does not, however, have to remain in total darkness because indoor light helps to inactivate the drug. The most frequent complications of PDT include injection site reaction, photosensitivity of the skin, and transient visual disturbance. The nurse should reassure the patient that the vision should return to its previous level in a few days (McGrory & Remington, 2004; Moshfeghi & Lewis, 2003; Smeltzer & Bare, 2004; Watkins, 2005).

Procedures Under Investigation

Macular Translocation

Macular translocation is an experimental surgical procedure in which a complete retinal detachment is created and functional sensory retina is moved away from areas of neovascularization into an area with a healthy retinal pigment epithelium. The choroidal neovascularization remains attached to the underlying retinal pigment epithelium. Laser can then be applied to the abnormal vessels, sparing the macula. Early reports have described preservation of vision and adverse effects, such as retinal detachment (Fine et al., 2000; Moshfeghi & Lewis, 2003).

Submacular Surgery

Submacular surgery is another experimental surgical procedure in which the choroidal neovascularization is mechanically removed with forceps and blood is extracted from the subretinal space surgically (Fine et al., 2000). Most data to date have come from small trials and shown marginal results (Arnold & Sarks, 2000). Large trials of the procedure have begun, and initial reports indicate that there is no difference in outcome between repeated laser photocoagulation and submacular surgery (Moshfeghi & Lewis, 2003). One multicenter trial showed little or no benefit to submacular surgery for persons with choroidal neovascularization, whose best corrected visual acuity was 20/100 or better. In this group, the risk of retinal detachment, recurrent neovascularization, and cataract outweighed the benefit of the surgery. There was, however, benefit for some older adults whose best corrected vision was worse than 20/100 (Hawkins et al., 2004).

Antiangiogenesis

Researchers have been studying blood vessel growth inhibitors to stop cancers. These growth inhibitors have potential for advances in the treatment of AMD. Abnormal angiogenesis occurs when cancer or other diseases, such as AMD, controls the normal process of angiogenesis. In eye disease, the abnormal blood vessels cause blindness, not the feeders of the disease, such as in cancer (Wilson, 2004). Investigations are being made into safe, effective drugs that can stop the growth of abnormal blood vessels (angiogenesis) in the choroid. Preclinical and early phase clinical trials are investigating thalidomide with and without laser photocoagulation. Other treatments being tested include a variety of antiangiogenic agents (anecortave acetate, triamcinolone acetonide) that are administered intravitreally or periocularly (Chopdar et al., 2003).

One large prospective randomized, double-blind, multicenter clinical trial investigated intravitreous injections of Pegaptanib, an antivascular endothelial growth factor in the treatment of neovascular AMD. Subjects who received eight to nine intraocular injections of the drug had better visual acuity at 54 weeks than controls who received sham injections. Serious side effects resulting in severe vision loss occurred in 0.1% of subjects, including endophthalmitis, traumatic injury to the lens, and retinal detachment (Gragoudas, Adamis, Cunningham, Feinsod, & Guyer, 2004).

Radiation

Early clinical trials of radiation therapy in AMD found that the treatment was ineffective in maintaining vision. A multicenter trial reported no difference in distance vision, but some benefit in near vision. The potential for benefit of radiation lies in the fact that proliferating vascular endothelial cells are especially sensitive to radiation. External-beam radiation destroys the neovascular areas and preserves the retinal vessels as they are relatively resistant to the radiation. It remains only a palliative measure, as complete destruction of the neovascularization is usually not possible (Fine et al., 2000; Moore, 2001). Subjects in a small clinical trial in the Netherlands showed a smaller decrease in visual acuity than untreated subjects after 1 year with radiation therapy (Fine et al.).

Retinal Prosthesis

Pilot feasibility studies have begun to evaluate the ability of a microchip implanted in the retina to produce artificial vision for people with severe retinal degeneration. There are many obstacles to the successful development of these prostheses. Currently there is no noninvasive method to determine the viability of retinal cells. The amount of electric current used to stimulate retinal cells and produce perception needs to be at a level that will not damage the retina or produce heat. The device must also be encapsulated so that it will not induce rejection, inflammation, or fibrosis. Most importantly, a successful interface between human neural tissue and electronic materials must be developed (Chopdar et al., 2003; Loewenstein, Montezuma, & Rizzo, 2004).

CONCLUSION

AMD can have a considerable effect on an older adult's health, functional ability, and quality of life. Nurses are in an excellent position to teach their patients measures to prevent or delay the onset of visual disability and to promote early identification of those who have the disease. Nurses should take a leadership role in helping older adults maintain independence, despite declining vision. Considerable medical research is being conducted related to vision loss and AMD. Little is available in the nursing literature, however, much of the care of older adults with AMD is within the scope of nursing practice. More research is necessary to validate the nurse's role in assisting the older adult with AMD to maintain function, adapt to the diagnosis of AMD, and to prevent disability.

REFERENCES

Age-Related Eye Diseases Study Research Group. (2001). A randomized, placebo-controlled, clinical trial of high-dose supplementation with vitamins C and E, beta carotene and zinc for age-related macular degeneration and vision loss: AREDS report no. 8. *Archives of Ophthalmology, 119*, 1417–1436.

Arnold, J. J., & Sarks, S. H. (2000). Age-related macular degeneration. *British Medical Journal, 321*, 741–744.

Chopdar, A., Chakravarthy, U., & Verma, D. (2003). Age related macular degeneration. *British Medical Jounal, 326,* 485–488.

Congdon, N., Friedman, D., & Lietman, T. (2003). Important causes of visual impairment in the world today. *Journal of the American Medical Association, 290,* 2057–2060.

Delcourt, C., Diaz, J. L., Ponton-Sanchez, A., & Papoz, L. (1998). Smoking and age-related macular degeneration. *Archives of Ophthalmology, 116*, 1031–1035.

Eye Diseases Prevalence Research Group. (2004). Causes and prevalence of visual impairment among adults in the United States. *Archives of Ophthalmology, 122,* 477–485.

Ferris, F. L., (2004). A new treatment for ocular neovascularization. *New England Journal of Medicine, 351*, 2863–2865.

Fine, S. L., Berger, J. W., Maguire, M. G., & Ho, A. C. (2000). Drug therapy: Age-related macular degeneration. *New England Journal of Medicine, 342*, 483–492.

Gragoudas, E. S., Adamis, A. P., Cunningham, E. T., Feinsod, M., & Guyer, D. R. (2004). Pegaptanib for neovascular age-related macular degeneration. *New England Journal of Medicine, 351,* 2805–2816.

Hall, N. F., Gale, C. R., Sydall, H., Phillips, D. I., & Marlyn, C. N. (2001). Risk of macular degeneration in users of statins: Cross sectional study. *British Medical Journal, 323*(7309), 375–376.

Hawkins, B. S., Bressler, N. M., Bresler, S. B., Davidorf, F. H., Hoskins. J. C., Marsh, M. J., et al. (2004). Surgical removal vs. observation for subfoveal choroidal neovascularization, either associated with the ocular histoplasmosis syndrome or idiopathic: I. ophthalmic findings from a randomized clinical trial: Submacular Surgery Trials (SST) Group H Trial: SST Report No. 9. *Archives of Ophthalmology, 122*(11), 1597–1612.

Loewenstein, J. I., Montezuma, S. R., & Rizzo, J. F. (2004). Outer retinal degeneration: An electronic retinal prosthesis as a treatment strategy. *Archives of Ophthalmology, 122*, 587–596.

Mares, J. A., LaRowe, T. L., & Blodi, B. A. (2004). Doctor, what vitamins should I take for my eyes? *Archives of Ophthalmology, 122*, 628–635.

McGrory, A., & Remington, R. (2004). Optimizing the functionality of clients with age-related macular degeneration. *Rehabilitation Nursing, 29*, 90–94.

Miller, C. A. (2004). *Nursing for wellness in older adults: Theory and practice*. Philadelphia: Lippincott Williams & Wilkins.

Moore, L. W. (2001). Macular degeneration in older adults. *Geriatric Nursing, 22*, 96–99.

Moshfeghi, D. M., & Lewis, H. (2003). Age-related macular degeneration: Evaluation and treatment. *Cleveland Clinic Journal of Medicine, 70*, 1017–1037.

Pache, M., Smeets, C., Gasio, P. F., Flammer, J., Wirz-Justice, A., & Kaiser, H. J. (2003). Colour vision deficiencies in Alzheimer's disease. *Age and Ageing, 32*, 422–426.

Rowe, S., MacLean, C. H., & Shekelle, P. (2004). Preventing visual loss from chronic eye disease in primary care: Scientific review. *Journal of the American Medical Association, 291*, 1487–1495.

Sadler, C. (2002). Limited vision. *Nursing Standard, 16*(42), 14–15.

Seddon, J. M., Cote, J., & Rosner, B. (2003). Progression of age-related macular degeneration: Association with dietary fat, transunsaturated fat, nuts, and fish intake. *Archives of Ophthalmology, 121*, 1728–1737.

Seddon, J. M., Willett, W. C., Speizer, F. E., & Hankinson, S. E. (1996). A prospective study of cigarette smoking and age-related macular degeneration in women. *Journal of the American Medical Association, 276*, 1141–1146.

Smeeding, S. (2001). Nutrition, supplements, and aging. *Geriatric Nursing.* 22(4), 219–224.

Smeltzer, S. C., & Bare, B. C. (2004). *Textbook of medical-surgical nursing.* Philadelphia: Lippincott Williams & Wilkins.

Tasman, W., & Rovner, B. (2004). Age-related macular degeneration: Treating the whole patient. *Archives of Ophthalmology, 122*, 648–649.

Tomany, S. C., Cruickshanks, K. J., Klein, R., Klein, B., & Knudtson, M. D. (2004). Sunlight and the 10 year incidence of age-related maculopathy: The Beaver Dam Eye Study. *Archives of Ophthalmology, 122*, 750–757.

Watkins, S. (2005). Visual impairment in older people: The nurse's role. *Nursing Standard, 19*(17), 45–55.

Wilson, J. F. (2004). Angiogenesis therapy moves beyond cancer. *Archives of Internal Medicine 141*(2), 165–168.

CHAPTER 3

Cataracts

Pat Gillett, Kate Goldblum, and Joyce Powers

A cataract is an opacity or change in color that occurs in the normally clear crystalline lens of the eye. The basic cause of visual impairment in patients with cataracts is impaired refractive ability of the cloudy lens, causing varying types and levels of visual disability. Without surgical intervention, cataracts can result in eventual blindness. Cataracts are very common in older adults. In those over age 75, visually significant cataracts occur in almost 40% of men and 46% of women. In the United States, cataract is the leading cause of reversible blindness in individuals over age 40. Worldwide, it is the leading cause of blindness in all individuals (Preferred Practice Patterns Committee [PPPC], Anterior Segment Panel, 2001; Solomon & Donnenfeld, 2003).

PATHOPHYSIOLOGY AND ETIOLOGY

Despite recognition of some risk factors as clearly implicated in cataract development, the underlying pathophysiology of cataract development is not fully understood. Current knowledge supports disruption in the lens proteins and a breakdown in homeostasis as part of the pathogenic process (Johns et al., 2001). Some of these disruptive processes occur predictably as a result of aging, but may also occur as the result of other factors. Both oxidative and photooxidative stress may play roles in cataract formation (Leske et al., 1998; Neale, Purdie, Hirst, & Green, 2003). Despite recognition of the role of oxidative damage in cataract development, current research provides no consistent information regarding the benefit of antioxidants in preventing cataract formation. Even studies that have shown some benefit have not clearly identified the specific antioxidants that may be helpful. These inconsistencies may reflect a multifactorial role of several antioxidants that must work together to protect the lens from oxidative damage (Age-Related Eye Disease Study [AREDS] Research Group, 2001; McNeil et al., 2004).

A well-known risk factor, diabetes, increases the risk of cataract formation by several possible mechanisms. When glucose levels are high, osmotic pressure results in lens swelling and opacification over the long term. Glycosylation of lens proteins increases the susceptibility of the lens to oxidation, eventually leading to cataract formation (Franke et al., 2003). Although aging is the primary risk factor for cataract development, there are many other implicated risk factors. In addition to diabetes, corticosteroid use and heavy smoking are also associated with higher rates of cataract development. Solar and other forms of ultraviolet radiation exposure, electrical shock, and intraocular inflammation are also associated with cataracts. Trauma, whether from blunt, penetrating, or surgical insults, predictably results in often-rapid formation of cataracts. In addition, cataracts occur in individuals with other hereditary diseases and certain systemic disorders, including galactosemia, myotonic dystrophy, hypocalcemia, and neurofibromatosis type II (Streeten, 2000).

SIGNS AND SYMPTOMS

The primary presenting symptom of individuals with cataracts is altered distant and/or near vision. Patients may complain of blurred or cloudy vision, glare, halos, difficulties with nighttime vision, or color distortion. Usually, the only sign of cataract is an observable lens opacity. However, an enlarged, cataractous lens may exert pressure on the iris, displacing it forward into the trabecular meshwork. This can subtly obstruct aqueous humor outflow and result in increased intraocular pressure. This pressure increase is generally small and has no subjective manifestations.

Health care practitioners can examine the crystalline lens of the eye directly. They may use several special instruments that provide light and magnification for viewing, such as the direct ophthalmoscope, indirect ophthalmoscope, or biomicroscope. These instruments allow visualization of cataracts, especially when the patient has a dilated pupil. Cataracts may be nuclear, cortical, posterior subcapsular, or any combination of these types. Anterior subcapsular cataracts represent a fourth category of cataract, but this type is uncommon. Anatomic location determines the type of cataract.

Nuclear cataracts are located in the lens nucleus and usually appear centrally on examination. They cause progressive myopia (nearsightedness) and have a characteristic brunescent (yellowish brown) quality that worsens over time. All individuals begin to lose the ability to focus on near objects about age 40 due to normal aging changes in the lens. These changes lead to lens inelasticity, preventing the lens from changing shape to alter the focal distance from distant objects to near objects, resulting in a condition called presbyopia. Presbyopic individuals sometimes notice an improved ability to see near objects without reading glasses as their cataracts cause progressive myopia, which compensates for their presbyopia. Thus, development of myopia secondary to nuclear cataracts partially restores the ability to see near objects without corrective lenses—older adults' "second sight." Nuclear cataracts usually affect distance vision to a greater extent than near vision. They are often slow to progress, but will eventually become completely opaque with a characteristic brunescent appearance.

Cortical cataracts are located in the lens cortex, so they may appear peripherally or centrally. These cataracts commonly cause complaints of glare and become white when mature and opaque. Posterior subcapsular cataracts (PSC) are located just anterior to the posterior capsule. They tend to affect near vision before distance vision, and younger individuals exhibit this type of cataract more often than nuclear or cortical opacities (PPPC, 2001). Anterior subcapsular cataracts are located between the lens capsule and the anterior lens epithelium. Anterior cataracts typically occur after trauma or uveitis (Goldblum, 2002).

Ophthalmologists often use one of several methods to quantify cataracts (Datiles, 1996). Some systems are quite subjective. Photographic quantification schemes and newer imaging techniques provide more objectivity, but variability in the visual needs of each patient limits the clinical usefulness of all methods.

DIAGNOSIS

Minimum Evaluation

A minimum evaluation to diagnose cataract and rule out other causes of visual impairment should include examination of the lens with slit lamp biomicroscopy and ophthalmoscopy, as well as a dilated ocular fundus examination and a gross assessment of visual fields and ocular motility. Determining the patient's best corrected visual acuity should include assessment of both near and distance acuities. Examination of the pupil and determination of the patient's intraocular pressure complete the minimum evaluation. It is important to measure intraocular pressure to determine whether the individual has glaucoma secondary to cataracts. Although it is uncommon, this condition can occur in patients with advanced cataracts. Phacomorphic glaucoma is an acute angle-closure disorder resulting from increased lens size. This condition predisposes the patient to pupillary block. Phacolytic glaucoma results when a hypermature cataract leaks lens substance causing open-angle glaucoma, secondary to phagocytes and free lens proteins in the anterior chamber (Cantor et al., 2001).

Additional Evaluation

Certain situations mandate additional evaluation. Testing for glare disability and contrast sensitivity may be necessary in a patient who does not demonstrate a significant loss of visual acuity, but has subjective complaints of difficulties related to visual disability. These patients may have debilitating glare or inability to continue their usual activities due to "eye strain." In patients with significant lens opacities or other obstructions of the ocular media that occlude the ocular fundus, other assessments may be necessary.

A potential acuity meter can assist in evaluating the patient's potential postoperative visual acuity. B-scan ultrasonography to rule out possible posterior pathology that could preclude a good surgical result may also be indicated. Additional testing may be needed to differentiate visual loss due to cataracts from other etiologies. Detailed visual field testing, electrooculogram, electroretinogram, and intravenous fluorescein angiography may all be indicated in certain situations. If the patient chooses to have surgery and has any actual or suspected corneal pathology, specular microscopy or corneal pachymetry can be helpful to identify problems prior to cataract surgery. Specular microscopy provides information on the status of the corneal endothelium. If the endothelium is already compromised, the intraocular manipulation that occurs with cataract extraction and intraocular lens implantation may further reduce the number of endothelial cells. Following surgery, the endothelial layer can become compromised enough to allow fluid into the stromal layer of the cornea and blisters may erupt from the epithelium on the corneal surface, resulting in a condition called bullous keratopathy. Pachymetry measures corneal thickness and can be useful in determining whether the cornea is edematous, indicating a potential problem.

MEDICAL AND SURGICAL MANAGEMENT

General Considerations

Determining optimal management for a patient with cataracts must include a careful history to determine whether the patient has a functional visual impairment, and if so, how severely it affects the patient's lifestyle. This information is imperative to determine appropriate treatment for each patient. Adequate vision for one patient may be completely intolerable for another, depending on the individual's visual needs. Patients are often vague about their functional impairments and it may be necessary to question them about the effect of their visual deficits on specific activities, including leisure pursuits. For example, careful questioning may reveal that the patient has largely replaced avid reading with other activities due to visual difficulties, or has quit driving at night due to incapacitating glare. In addition, cataracts usually develop slowly and patients often do not recognize the significant declines that have occurred over time. The older adult's family can be a valuable source of information. Family members may notice changes such as a recently increased number of falls or inability to confidently navigate steps. Although the evidence is contradictory, subtle cognitive changes may be related to visual impairment secondary to cataracts (Grodstein, Chen, & Hankinson, 2003; Tamura et al., 2004). A thorough history focusing on the patient's prior and current activities may be the only way to obtain this information. Using a questionnaire to elicit specific information to identify and assess functional visual disability specific to the older adult's desired or needed activities can be very useful. One commonly used questionnaire to measure functional impairment is the VF-14 (Steinberg et al., 1994).

Medical Management

When an older adult has a cataract causing some level of visual impairment, the individual may assume surgery is the only alternative. However, appropriate information about nonsurgical options, combined with a careful visual history, will help guide the older adult in making an informed decision about whether surgery is the best option. Individuals with a cataract should understand that cataract surgery is almost always an elective procedure, necessary only if the level of vision provided by an optimal spectacle correction does not allow adequate functioning. A good spectacle correction can help compensate for any myopia induced by the cataract. A stronger bifocal in the spectacle or some other form of magnification may be adequate to improve near vision to a level acceptable to the individual. Some older adults are able to modify their lifestyle to accommodate visual impairment due to cataract. The amount of accommodation acceptable or possible for each person will vary, but many individuals may not want to compromise their lifestyles. However, stronger ambient lighting may allow comfortable reading, and forgoing nighttime driving may obviate the need for surgery, at least temporarily. Older adults should understand that such measures are palliative and the cataract will continue to worsen, although progression may occur very gradually. Each individual should have enough information to be confident that postponing surgical treatment is a valid option, depending on his or her visual needs.

Surgical Management

Indications and Contraindications

The primary indication for surgical extraction is visual impairment unacceptably limiting the ability to engage in usual and desired activities. A secondary indication is inability to visualize the ocular fundus in order to monitor or treat other conditions such as diabetic retinopathy, macular degeneration, or glaucoma. Rarely, the presence of lens-induced inflammation or glaucoma may mandate a surgical approach. Although the risk of complications is very low with cataract surgery (usually 5% or less), older adults should have appropriate information so they can weigh the potential risks against the potential benefits. The risk/benefit ratio is altered in one-eyed patients. One-eyed individuals are those who are blind or have no useful vision in one eye, as well as those who are actually missing one eye. Health care providers and one-eyed individuals need to understand that although the risk of vision loss from cataract surgery is minimal, *any* loss could be catastrophic in a one-eyed patient. Imperfect vision may be more acceptable in this situation.

The primary contraindication to surgical removal of a cataract is that the individual does not want surgery. Surgery is also not indicated if the older adult's vision is adequately improved with medical measures, such as stronger spectacles or increased ambient lighting. Other contraindications include an incompetent patient when there is no legal representative available to give informed consent, or lack of reasonable expectation of improved vision following surgery. In addition, surgery is contraindicated if the patient is medically unable to undergo surgery or will not have access to necessary postoperative care (PPPC, 2001).

Choice of Anesthesia

Current surgical management is almost exclusively an outpatient procedure employing some form of local anesthesia (topical, retrobulbar, peribulbar, periocular, or intracameral). This minimizes the risks of anesthesia, especially for older patients who often have co-morbidities. The type of anesthesia is determined primarily by patient considerations and surgeon preference. The patient's level of anxiety, general health status, and the presence of specific co-morbidities may affect anesthesia choice (Goldblum, 2002). Disorders such as

Parkinsonism, conditions requiring anticoagulant therapy, or dementia may all influence the decision.

Preoperative Preparation

The appropriate preoperative evaluation for older adults planning to have cataract extraction varies from patient to patient. In addition, many surgical facilities have different requirements. Based on specific individual needs, some patients may need medical testing such as electrolytes or electrocardiogram (ECG). However, most patients do not need preoperative testing prior to cataract surgery. In one large study, preoperative testing (ECG, complete blood count, electrolytes, urea nitrogen, creatinine, and glucose) did not reduce the incidence of intraoperative or postoperative medical events or rate of complications (Schein et al., 2000).

All patients should be asked about a focused history, including a review of systems, and a physical examination pertinent to their individual situation and risk factors should be performed (PPPC, 2001). Past and current health status and conditions, medications, allergies, and previous surgeries are relevant information. It is prudent to measure the patient's blood pressure during the preoperative visit to identify undiagnosed hypertension or hypertension not well-controlled on current medication. If this is a problem, it should be addressed prior to surgery. In addition to this general medical assessment and the complete ophthalmic examination discussed previously, additional measurements of corneal curvature and axial length of the eye are necessary for calculation of the appropriate intraocular lens power.

Older adults need appropriate education prior to surgery. They should receive verbal and written preoperative and postoperative instructions. Printed information should use a standard type face large enough to see easily. Because about half the adults in the United States read at or below the eighth-grade reading level (Nickel, 2003), printed material should not exceed this level of difficulty. Appropriate instruction prior to surgery includes information about preoperative fasting requirements and medication use as well as postoperative care including eye drops, permissible activity, and recommended follow-up.

Surgical Procedures

Extracapsular cataract extraction (ECCE) is currently the most common type of cataract surgery and may be performed either using phacoemulsification or without using phacoemulsification. Cataract extraction by phacoemulsification (CEPE) is the method of extracapsular surgery most ophthalmologists

use. Most surgeons also implant an intraocular lens (IOL) in the capsular bag or in the ciliary sulcus in front of a partially intact capsular bag at
the time of cataract extraction (PPPC, 2001). In both types of extracapsular
cataract extraction (ECCE without phacoemulsification and CEPE), the surgeon makes a small opening in the anterior part of the capsule surrounding
the lens and removes the lens nucleus, leaving the rest of the capsule intact. In ECCE without phacoemulsification, the surgeon manually removes
the nucleus with a lens loop and then removes cortical fragments with an irri-
gation/aspiration instrument. In CEPE, the surgeon uses a phacoemulsification
unit to deliver ultrasonic power through a cannulated tip. The tip fragments
the lens nucleus and removes the fragments with suction while maintaining
the intraocular space with concurrent irrigation of balanced salt solution. Removal of the remaining cortex is similar to the procedure used in standard
ECCE.

Intracapsular cataract extraction (ICCE) has been largely relegated to special circumstances such as subluxation or dislocation of the lens (Johns et al.,
2001). In contrast to extracapsular extraction, in ICCE the surgeon removes the
entire lens, including the capsule. This is accomplished by using a cryotherapy
tip, which forms an ice ball when applied to the lens surface and allows intact
removal of the lens. Intraocular lens (IOL) placement following an intracapsular procedure is usually in the anterior chamber because no capsular bag is
present. The surgeon may alternatively choose to suture a posterior chamber
lens to the sclera when there is no capsular support.

Older adults sometimes have the mistaken impression that cataract
surgery can be done with laser. This misunderstanding usually results from
the fact that the posterior capsule, left intact following extracapsular cataract
surgery, can become opaque weeks to years following cataract extraction. In
this case, a laser procedure using the neodymium yttrium-aluminum-garnet
(Nd:YAG) laser will make an opening in the cloudy posterior capsule. Because
the posterior capsule opacity is often called a "secondary cataract," patients
may conclude that cataracts can be removed with laser.

Complications

Cataract surgery may be complicated by adverse events at any time during
the perioperative period. However, major complications occur in less than 4%
of patients overall. Ninety-five percent of patients without preexisting ocular
problems will achieve visual acuity of 20/40 or better (PPPC, 2001). Patients
with other ocular problems who have cataract surgery have an increased risk
of complications. Increased risks associated with the preoperative presence of
diabetic retinopathy include macular edema, vitreous hemorrhage, intraocular

inflammation, and endophthalmitis. Preexisting glaucoma, intraocular inflammation, or macular degeneration also increase the risk of complications.

A preoperative complication may arise from the retrobulbar injection of anesthesia. The injection may puncture the globe or deliver the anesthetic into the optic nerve or extraocular muscles. Especially in anti-coagulated patients, it may also result in retrobulbar hemorrhage. Intraoperatively, the capsule may rupture, resulting in possible loss of nuclear or cortical fragments into the vitreous. Capsular rupture may also result in vitreous moving forward into the anterior chamber and possibly into the wound. Although very rare in phacoemulsification procedures, expulsive choroidal hemorrhage is a devastating complication (Steinert et al., 2000). The hemorrhage increases pressure inside the eye, which can cause the intraocular contents to prolapse through the surgical wound.

Postoperatively, the primary early complication is endophthalmitis, a potentially devastating and generalized infection of all the ocular tissues. Fortunately, it occurs very rarely (Goldblum, 2002). Other potential complications that occur later in the postoperative period include cystoid macular edema, dislocation of the IOL, retinal detachment, corneal problems, diplopia, or ptosis. The most frequent postoperative complication is posterior capsule opacity. However, as noted previously this complication is easily treated by opening the posterior capsule with laser.

Postoperative Considerations

Most patients leave the surgical facility following cataract surgery within 1 to 3 hours. Complications that may delay discharge or require hospitalization include pulmonary or cardiovascular problems, alterations in mental status, uncontrolled blood glucose levels, severe pain, hyphema, or expulsive hemorrhage.

Postoperative medications usually include topical antibiotic and anti-inflammatory agents. Most patients will have few activity restrictions, depending on their surgeon's preference. The first follow-up visit is usually within 1 to 2 days after surgery and the second follow-up examination 4 to 7 days after surgery (PPPC, 2001). The frequency and timing of subsequent examinations depend on the patient's condition. A final visit for postoperative refraction usually occurs 4 weeks postoperatively, but may be sooner.

Postoperative Visual Rehabilitation

Implantation of IOLs at the time of cataract extraction has revolutionized postoperative visual rehabilitation following cataract extraction, almost completely replacing use of cataract spectacles and aphakic contact lenses except in unusual circumstances. Cataract spectacles have high-magnification lenses, necessary to compensate for removal of the eye's natural lens. An individual who wears this type of spectacle must learn to turn her or his head to look at objects directly because of the distortion induced when looking through the periphery of the lenses. In addition, objects appear about 30% larger through these lenses, even on direct gaze. Aphakic contact lenses do not share these undesirable optical properties, but are difficult for many older patients to manipulate, often are not well tolerated, and require a significant healing time before patients can begin wearing them.

IOL implantation provides immediate visual rehabilitation, although many patients still require at least some additional spectacle correction to maximize distance visual acuity. This is particularly true of patients who have significant corneal astigmatism, because most IOLs implanted today do not correct astigmatism. Despite some availability of multifocal IOLs to correct presbyopia, problems with these IOLs remain and most patients also need postoperative spectacle correction for good near vision (Nijkamp et al., 2004).

SUMMARY

Cataracts are a common occurrence with aging and are nearly ubiquitous in the very old, making this cause of vision loss a significant concern for nurses who provide care to older adults. Understanding the disease process, indications and contraindications for surgery, and the medical and surgical management of cataracts will allow nurses to provide appropriate patient education. Older adults need to know that the safety and efficacy of modern cataract surgery make it unnecessary to compromise independence and lifestyle because of vision loss secondary to a cataract. At the same time, an understanding that the simple presence of a cataract does not mandate surgery is also important. Nurses who provide care to older adults in any setting are ideally suited to assess the impact of vision loss resulting from cataracts on the lives of their patients. Providing accurate information will help patients make a truly informed decision about the management options. Rapidly occurring advances in cataract surgery and IOL design mandate constant learning to remain informed in order to provide a high level of care to patients with cataracts.

REFERENCES

Age-Related Eye Disease Study Research Group. (2001). A randomized, placebo-controlled, clinical trial of high-dose supplementation with vitamins C and E and beta carotene for age-related cataract and vision loss: AREDS report no. 9. *Archives of Ophthalmology, 119,* 1439–1452.

Cantor, L., Fechtner, R. D., Michael, A. J., Simmons, S. T., Wilson, M. R., & Brown, S. V. L. (2001). *Basic and clinical science course: Glaucoma.* San Francisco: The Foundation of the American Academy of Ophthalmology.

Datiles, M. B., III (1996). Clinical evaluation of cataracts. In W. Tasman & E. A. Jaeger (Eds.), *Duane's clinical ophthalmology, Vol. 1* (Rev. ed., pp. 1–15). Philadelphia: Lippincott-Raven.

Franke, S., Dawczynski, J., Strobel, J., Niwa, T., Stahl, P., & Stein, G. (2003). Increased levels of advanced glycation end products in human cataractous lenses. *Journal of Cataract and Refractive Surgery, 29*(5), 998–1004.

Goldblum, K. (2002). Lens disorders. In K. Goldblum & P. A. Lamb (Eds.), *Core curriculum for ophthalmic nursing* (2nd ed., pp. 243–263). Dubuque, IA: Kendall/Hunt Publishing Company.

Grodstein, F., Chen, J., & Hankinson, S. E. (2003). Cataract extraction and cognitive function in older women. *Epidemiology, 14*(4), 493–497.

Johns, K. G., Feder, R. S., Hamill, M. B., Miller-Meeks, M. J., Rosenfeld, S. I., & Perry, P. E. (2001). *Basic and clinical science course: Lens and cataract.* San Francisco: Foundation of the American Academy of Ophthalmology.

Leske, M. C., Chylack, L. T., Jr., He, Q., Wu, S. Y., Schoenfeld, E., Friend, J., & Wolfe, J. (1998). Antioxidant vitamins and nuclear opacities: The longitudinal study of cataract. *Ophthalmology, 105*(5), 831–836.

McNeil, J. J., Robman, L., Tikellis, G., Sinclair, M. I., McCarty, C. A., & Taylor, H. R. (2004). Vitamin E supplementation and cataract: Randomized controlled trial. *Ophthalmology, 111*(1), 75–84.

Neale, R. E., Purdie, J. L., Hirst, L. W., & Green, A. C. (2003). Sun exposure as a risk factor for nuclear cataract. *Epidemiology, 14*(6), 707–712.

Nickel, M. (2003). *Fourth annual 'e-government' survey: Readability is a problem for state and federal government Web sites.* Retrieved February 13, 2005, from http://www.brown.edu/Administration/News_Bureau/2003-04/03-025.html

Nijkamp, D. D., Dolders, M. G., de Brabander, J., van den Borne, B., Hendrikse, F., & Nuijts, R. M. (2004). Effectiveness of multifocal intraocular lenses to correct presbyopia after cataract surgery: A randomized controlled trial. *Ophthalmology, 111*(10), 1832–1839.

Preferred Practice Patterns Committee [PPPC], Anterior Segment Panel. (2001). *Preferred practice pattern: Cataract in the adult eye.* San Francisco: American Academy of Ophthalmology.

Schein, O. D., Katz, J., Bass, E. B., Tielsch, J. M., Lubomski, L. H., Feldman, M. A., et al. (2000). The value of routine preoperative medical testing before cataract surgery. *New England Journal of Medicine, 342*, 168–175.

Solomon, R., & Donnenfeld, E. D. (2003). Recent advances and future frontiers in treating age-related cataracts. *Journal of the American Medical Association, 290*(2), 248–251.

Steinberg, E. P., Tielsch, J. M., Schein, O. D., Javitt, J. C., Sharkey, P. Cassard, S. D., et al. (1994). The VF-14. An index of functional impairment in patients with cataract. *Archives of Ophthalmology, 112*, 630–638.

Steinert, R. F., Cionni, R. J., Osher, R. H., Blumenkranz, M. S., Koch, D. D., Novak, K. D., et al. (2000). Complications of cataract surgery. In D. M. Albert & F. A. Jakobiec (Eds.), *Principles and practice of ophthalmology* (2nd ed., Chapter 110) [CD-ROM]. Philadelphia: Saunders.

Streeten, B. W. (2000). Pathology of the lens. In D. M. Albert & F. A. Jakobiec (Eds.), *Principles and practice of ophthalmology* (2nd ed., Chapter 272) [CD-ROM]. Philadelphia: Saunders.

Tamura, H., Tsukamoto, H., Mukai, S., Kato, T., Minamoto, A., Ohno, Y., et al. (2004). Improvement in cognitive impairment after cataract surgery in elderly patients. *Journal of Cataract and Refractive Surgery, 30*(3), 598–602.

CHAPTER 4

Glaucoma

Arlene McGrory

Glaucoma is the second most frequent cause of vision impairment and legal blindness among older adults in the United States and the leading cause of blindness for African Americans. About 120,000 people in the United States are blind because of glaucoma (American Academy of Ophthalmology [AAO], 2002). There is no known cure, and the primary treatment modality is eye medications for the duration of one's life. Glaucoma can cause disability, limitation of functioning, and decreased quality of life in older adults. With increased visual disability, falls and fractures may cause hospital or nursing home admission and premature death in the older adult population (Desai, Pratt, Lentzner, & Robinson, 2001).

Glaucoma can occur at any time in the life cycle. It is more common in older adults, however, and 3% of those over 55 years of age have glaucoma (Distelhorst & Hughes, 2003). There has been a 3% increase in glaucoma from 1984 to 1995 in noninstitutionalized older adults. Those who are nearsighted have an increased chance of developing glaucoma. It is also more common in Black older adults than in White older adults. Fifteen percent of Black older adults have glaucoma in contrast to 7% of those older adults who are White. Fifty percent of those who have glaucoma are not aware that they have the condition (Desai et al., 2001).

There are two major types of glaucoma: open-angle and angle-closure. Open-angle glaucoma is the most common form of glaucoma. It is usually asymptomatic, that is, without pain. Angle-closure glaucoma, the least common form of glaucoma, is also called "narrow-angle" or "acute glaucoma." Primary angle-closure glaucoma (PACG) can be acute or it can occur painlessly and asymptomatically over a longer time frame (Wilensky & Campbell, 2000).

DIAGNOSIS

Intraocular Pressure

Glaucoma has been traditionally defined as increased intraocular pressure (IOP) beyond the normal pressure range of 10 to 21 mm Hg. As many as one-half of patients with open-angle glaucoma have normal IOP, however (AAO, 2002; Distelhorst & Hughes, 2003). A patient with increased IOP and no evidence of optic nerve damage is called a glaucoma suspect (AAO, 2002). Elevated IOP is a modifiable risk factor in open-angle glaucoma, but it is not diagnostic of the condition (Distelhorst & Hughes). Angle-closure glaucoma may or may not be associated with elevated IOP (AAO, 2000b), but when it is elevated it occurs in proportion to the degree of angle closure (Wilensky & Campbell, 2000).

Optic Neuropathy

In open-angle glaucoma, optic cup changes can precede visual field changes (AAO, 2003). Diagnosis of open-angle glaucoma is confirmed by dividing the diameter of the outside cup by the inside ring; the result is expressed as a fraction or a decimal. It is not expressed as a ratio. A patient with glaucoma has a symmetrically enlarged cup-to-disc ratio greater than 0.5, an asymmetrical cup-to-disc ratio between the eyes of 0.2 or greater, or an optic nerve cup that is highly asymmetric in one eye (Distelhorst & Hughes, 2003). There may be notching of the disc rim, with abnormalities in retinal nerve fibers that are suggestive of a loss of nerve tissue (AAO). During an attack of acute angle-closure glaucoma, the optic nerve becomes congested followed by pallor and atrophy, without much cupping. With chronic angle-closure glaucoma, there is a slowly enlarging optic cup, with loss of neuroretinal rim tissue (Wilensky & Campbell, 2000).

Visual Field Defects

Visual field defects are noted with open-angle and angle-closure glaucoma. Peripheral vision loss is at first subtle. Usually the patient notices the visual field loss when the condition is well advanced. The severity of the damage from glaucoma can be ascertained by determining visual field abnormalities. The patient with mild open-angle glaucoma may have optic nerve changes but a normal visual field. Moderate glaucoma is present if there are visual field changes in one hemifield. Open-angle glaucoma is severe if there are changes in both hemifields (AAO, 2003). Scotoma, reduced vision in an otherwise normal visual field, can occur in a variety of patterns with glaucoma. The primary technique for evaluating visual field is automated perimetry. For the patient with acute angle-closure glaucoma, the visual fields are assessed after emergency treatment.

PATHOPHYSIOLOGY AND RISK FACTORS

Increased IOP may be caused by either an increase in the production of aqueous humor at the ciliary body, or a diminished outflow of aqueous humor from the eye at the canal of Schlemm. The normal pathway for aqueous humor outflow is through the anterior chamber to the trabecular meshwork, canal of Schlemm, capillaries, and systemic circulation. A decrease in the outflow of aqueous humor through the pathway results in an increase in intraocular pressure. Increased IOP has adverse effects on vision, as it causes ischemia and atrophy of the optic nerve, and may result in irreversible blindness, if not detected and treated effectively.

Glaucoma may be either primary or secondary. Primary glaucoma exists without other co-morbid problems. Secondary glaucoma occurs as a result of another problem, such as a tumor, surgery, recurrent ocular inflammation, or the use of steroids. Patients with diabetes may have an increased risk of developing glaucoma (AAO, 2000a). There are contradictory findings about the prevalence of diabetes in open-angle glaucoma patients. Some studies have linked diabetes to the development of open-angle glaucoma (AAO, 2002), and other studies have found that the presence of diabetes may have a protective effect in the development of primary open-angle glaucoma (POAG) (Gordon et al., 2002). Other risk factors that have been associated with the development of glaucoma include low diastolic perfusion pressures (diastolic blood pressure (BP) subtracted from IOP) and the presence of migraine headaches and peripheral vasospasm (AAO, 2003).

Open-Angle Glaucoma

Open-angle glaucoma results from loss of retinal ganglion cells, atrophy of the optic nerve, and enlargement of the optic nerve cup. Changes in the optic nerve or retinal nerve fiber may occur before there is evidence of measurable visual field defects. Hemorrhages may be noted around the optic nerve head before visual field changes (AAO, 2003).

The risk factors for the development of POAG include increasing intraocular pressure, Black race, first-degree relative with glaucoma, older age, and central corneal thickness. Increasing IOP has been shown to cause optic nerve damage. Race is a very important factor in the development of open-angle glaucoma. Blindness in African Americans with glaucoma occurs four to eight times as often as in White Americans, and it occurs at a younger age in Black Americans (AAO, 2003). The reason is unknown. Family history of glaucoma in a sibling or other first-degree relative increases the risk of developing open-angle glaucoma (AAO, 2000a).

Angle-Closure Glaucoma

In angle-closure glaucoma, the iris slides forward closing off the normal open angle, blocking the pupil, and occluding the flow of aqueous humor from the trabecular meshwork. The intraocular pressure increases to a dangerous level of 60 to 80 mm Hg (Wilensky & Campbell, 2000). There are several factors that put the patient at risk for angle-closure glaucoma. Patients with small eyes, hyperopia (short axial eye length), or who have a smaller anterior chamber, have an increased susceptibility to angle-closure glaucoma. With aging, the lens enlarges and can push the iris forward, thereby increasing the chance of angle-closure glaucoma. Other risk factors are a family history of angle closure, being an older adult, female gender, and Eskimo or Far Eastern Asian ethnicity (AAO, 2000a). Miotic medications can cause an attack of angle-closure glaucoma because the medication causes the lens to move forward and block the angle. Excessive reading with its increased accommodative effort can also cause an attack of angle-closure glaucoma (Wilensky & Campbell).

Pathologic changes that may occur after an episode of acute angle-closure glaucoma include corneal edema, necrosis of the iris, synechiae (adhesions of cornea and iris) formation, cataracts, and temporary ciliary body hyposecretion. Optic nerve edema can temporarily or permanently reduce vision (Wilensky & Campbell, 2000). Glaukomflecken is the development of irregular, sometimes star-shaped, changes in the lens after an attack of acute angle-closure glaucoma. These changes are visible in the irregularly mid-dilated and fixed pupil (Wilensky & Campbell). The pathologic changes that may result from chronic angle-closure glaucoma include gradual enlargement of the optic cup and a diminished visual field. Changes in the trabecular meshwork may also occur.

SIGNS AND SYMPTOMS OF GLAUCOMA

Open-angle glaucoma is largely asymptomatic. The older adult may complain of headaches or achy pains behind the eye and may note a gradual reduction in near vision. Upon ophthalmic exam there may be an abnormal optic disc, nerve fiber layer defect, a visual field defect, or elevated intraocular pressure. Vision may be diminished later in the disease.

During the crisis of acute closed-angle glaucoma, the client usually looks ill and complains of sudden onset of unilateral ocular pain that radiates to the forehead. Nausea and vomiting often ensues. The client often reports seeing halos around lights and has a red sclera. The cornea may become steamy and edematous from increased IOP causing fluid to leak into the cornea from the anterior chamber (Wilensky & Campbell, 2000). The pupil dilates slowly. The onset of an episode can occur after the pupil is dilated from mydriatic medications, systemic medications that dilate the pupil, severe stress, or being in a dark room resulting in partial dilation of the pupil (Wilensky & Campbell).

EARLY DETECTION OF GLAUCOMA

Early detection and treatment of glaucoma can delay impairments and preserve vision. For adults with no risk factors, the AAO (2000a) recommends a complete vision exam at least once during the 20s, at least twice during the 30s, every 2 to 4 years from age 40 to 64, and every 1 to 2 years for everyone 65 years and older.

Diabetics with an onset after 30 years of age without retinopathy should have an eye exam annually (AAO, 2000a). Those who have an onset of diabetes before the age of 30 without retinopathy should have an eye exam 5 years after onset and then yearly. Diabetics considering pregnancy should have a complete eye examination prior to conception. An alternative would be to have an eye examination early in the first trimester and every 3 months.

Patients with risk factors for glaucoma, for example, persons of African descent or who have a family history of glaucoma, should have more frequent eye exams. During the 20s the eyes should be examined every 3 to 5 years; from 30 to 64 years, every 2 to 4 years; and after 65 years, every 1 to 2 years (AAO, 2000a).

Undiagnosed vision problems in older adults can result in falls, inability to self-administer medications, difficulty understanding and following directions, and states of confusion. The nurse's role during a focused eye exam is to be alert to those individuals who are especially at risk. The nurse should also take an active role in the performance of vision screening and should initiate referrals to an ophthalmologist. To facilitate the process of the eye health exam with an older person who may be visually impaired, shake hands with the person and orient the person to the surroundings of the examining room. Allowing the older person to wear glasses will help communication (Bickley, 2003).

Focused Health History in an Older Adult With Glaucoma

The components of a focused health history are reviewed in this section to facilitate history taking by the nurse caring for the older adult.

Chief Complaint

The older adult should be asked why he or she is seeking treatment. POAG and chronic narrow-angle glaucoma can be present without any symptoms. There may be complaints of aching eyes. Kappes and McNair (2003) recommend that the presence of headache and visual changes should alert the nurse to consider the possibility of glaucoma.

A brief overview of general health should be obtained.

Biographical Data

In obtaining biographical information, the nurse should be alert to the possibility of glaucoma in older adults and any person of Black heritage. In addition, the patient should be asked about the history of smoking, alcohol use, and occupation.

Past Health History

A history of ocular disease, ocular injury, myopia, or steroid use should be noted. In addition, the presence of diabetes mellitus, cardiac or respiratory disease should be determined. Medications usually given for glaucoma, in particular, beta-blocker eye drops (Table 4.1), may have adverse effects on a patient with a cardiac or respiratory condition.

Family History

Because glaucoma may occur more commonly in first-degree relatives, it is important to note whether glaucoma is present in any first-degree relatives.

Allergy

Allergies to medications can preclude their use with glaucoma. Anyone with an allergy to sulfa should not be treated with acetazolamide (Table 4.2). All medication allergies should be identified.

TABLE 4.1 Beta-Blockers

(Beta-adrenergic Antagonists)

Name/Dose	Action/Use	Caution/Side Effects	Nursing Concerns
Timolol maleate (Timoptic) 0.1%, 0.25%, 0.5% 1 drop once or twice daily (most common form available)	Action: Noncardioselective beta 1 and beta 2 blockers reduces the aqueous humor production Does not cause pupillary constriction, change in accommodation, night blindness or blurred vision Use: open-angle and acute angle-closure glaucoma	May be absorbed systemically Contraindicated in bronchial asthma, chronic obstructive pulmonary disease (COPD), sinus bradycardia, second & third degree AV block, cardiac failure, and cardiogenic shock May mask signs of hypoglycemia in diabetics	When used to reduce IOP in angle-closure glaucoma, use with a miotic To reverse the effects of beta-blockers, use beta agonists (isoproterenol, dopamine, dobutamine, and norepinephrine)
Bexatolol (Betoptic S) 0.25%, 0.5% 1 drop twice a day	Action: Cardioselective less potent than timolol Use: ocular hypertension and chronic open-angle glaucoma		Shake suspension well

Sources: American Society of Health-System Pharmacists (2003). *AHFS Drug Handbook* (2nd ed.); Philadelphia, PA: Lippincott Williams & Wilkins. Facts and Comparisons (2005). Agents for glaucoma. *Drug facts and comparisons 2006* (pp. 2255–2276). St. Louis, MO: Wolters Kluwer Health.

TABLE 4.2 Carbonic Anhydrase Inhibitors (CAIs)

Name/Dose	Action/Use	Caution/Side Effects	Nursing Concerns
Dorzolamide (Trusopt) 2% 1 drop every 8 hours	Action: same action as below Uses: open-angle glaucoma	Ocular: burning, stinging, foreign body sensation Systemic; bitter taste	All CAIs—caution in patient allergic to sulfonamides All sulfonamides may cause rash and more severe reactions. Co-administration of dorzolamide and acetazolamide is not recommended.
Acetazolamide (Diamox) oral: 250 mg to 1 g of immediate release in divided doses per day or sustained release capsule 500 mg twice a day IV: up to 500 mg in 100 ml of D5W or NS. Infuse over 30 minutes	Action: inhibits carbonic anhydrase and reduces aqueous humor rate resulting in decrease IOP Use: adjunctive treatment of glaucoma in acute situations, not for chronic treatment Caution in COPD	Can cause blood dyscrasias, numbness, and tingling of extremities and perioral area, fatigue, GI irritation, diarrhea, nausea. Contraindicated: liver disease, renal disease, and kidney stones	30%–80% of patients cannot tolerate the side effects that limit chronic use. Avoid long-term use. Potential for excessive diuresis Monitor electrolytes Acetazolamide alkalizes urine, and this may decrease excretion of some drugs (amphetamines, procainamide, quinidine). Increased excretion of lithium and phenobarbital may require dose adjustments.
Methazolamide (Nepthzane) 25–100 mg two or three times a day	Action: same as acetazolamide Produces less acidosis and parasthesia than acetazolamide Uses: same as acetazolamide		

Sources: Bartlett, J. D., Jaanus, S. D., Fiscella, R. G., & Sharir, M. (2001). Ocular hypotensive drugs. In J. D. Bartlett and S. D. Jaanus (Eds.), *Clinical ocular pharmacology* (4th ed., pp. 167–218). Boston, MA: Butterworth-Heinemann.
Lacy, C. F., Armstrong, L. L., Goldman, M. P., & Lance, L. L. (2005). *Lexi-Comp's drug information handbook* (13th ed.). Hudson, OH: Lexi-Comp.

Functional Health Exam

A typical day for the patient should be described. Some of the questions that may be asked include: What are the normal activities of daily living? Have there been any changes in the ability to carry out these activities? Have family relationships changed because of declining vision? Have normal activities been curtailed recently because of vision difficulties? Does the older adult drive? Does the individual do any close work like reading, computer use, or television viewing; or does the individual have any other hobbies requiring close work? Is there any change in the ability to do close work? Are there any recent falls? What is the normal exercise pattern? Does the older adult get sufficient sleep, or does eye pain interfere? Does the occupation of the older adult put eye health at risk? Are protective glasses worn? Are recreational drugs used? The identification of drug use is important because recreational drugs can dilate or constrict pupils and can therefore affect drainage of aqueous fluid.

Psychosocial profile is important because it reflects coping abilities, roles, relationships, and personal habits.

All medications should be reviewed including ophthalmic, systemic, over-the-counter, and herbal medications.

Review of Systems

HEENT. Current visual acuity and any recent changes in acuity with or without glasses or contact lenses should be noted. A history of headaches, head injury, ocular injury, eye surgery, myopia, or steroid use should be identified. Kappes and McNair (2003) emphasize the importance of thoroughly investigating any complaint of headache and considering the possibility that the headache may be eye related. Changes in vision may be an early sign of increased intraocular pressure. The most recent eye exam should be recorded.

Respiratory. A history of chronic obstructive pulmonary disease should be determined, because it may preclude the use of beta-blockers in treatment of glaucoma.

Cardiovascular. A history of hypertension or other cardiovascular problem should be described. A history of cardiac problems may preclude use of beta-blockers in treating glaucoma. In addition, cardiovascular problems may occur concurrently with retinal changes and damage to the optic nerve, as well as decreased visual field.

Gastrointestinal. A history of liver disease should be identified, because the liver is essential in the metabolism of many medications.

Genitourinary. Renal problems may impair the excretion of medications and should be considered when prescribing medications for those with glaucoma.

Neurological. Neurological problems that affect vision may cause the older adult to seek health care. Multiple sclerosis can affect the optic nerve. Myasthenia gravis may cause ptosis and therefore impair vision. Trigeminal neuralgia may cause orbital pain (Dillon, 2003).

Endocrine. Determining whether an older adult has diabetes mellitus is important. Those with diabetes may have an increased chance of developing glaucoma.

Eye Examination for the Detection of Glaucoma

The following section describes the eye examination that the nurse should perform with those older adults being assessed for the presence of glaucoma. Glaucoma may be suspected on the basis of the results of an eye examination.

General Survey

The overall appearance of the older adult should be inspected. The patient's orientation and general mental status should be noted. Visual defects and gross eye abnormalities, like ptosis or exophthalmos, should be recorded. Blood pressure is important because it can alert the nurse to possible abnormal findings during fundoscopic examination.

Visual Acuity

Each eye should be tested for visual acuity individually, followed by testing of vision of both eyes together. The patient should begin by covering one eye and then covering the opposite eye while reading the vision chart. Testing should be performed first without corrective lenses and then with correction. To test distance vision, the Snellen chart should be used at a distance of 20 feet. Vision is recorded as the smallest line of print that can be read with no more than two incorrect answers. The Snellen E chart is used for individuals who do not know the alphabet, are illiterate, or are non-English-speaking. To test near vision, the Jaeger card is read at a distance of 14 inches. Alternately, a newspaper can be used and the distance from the eye where the print can be read clearly is recorded.

Color Vision

Defects in color vision are not usually associated with glaucoma. The Ishihara cards or colored bars on the Snellen eye chart can be used to evaluate color vision.

Visual Fields

Evaluation of the visual field is the mainstay of diagnosis and assists in the management of glaucoma (Distelhorst & Hughes, 2003). POAG can result in a loss of peripheral vision. Peripheral vision is measured in the horizontal, vertical, superior, inferior, medial (nasal), and lateral (temporal) fields of gaze. The nurse should ask the patient to look with both eyes directly into the nurse's eyes. As the examiner returns the patient's gaze, the nurse's index finger should be held lateral to the ear and moved from the periphery to the center of the visual field in order to test the lateral field of gaze (Bickley, 2003). The patient should be asked to say "now" when the finger comes into view (Dillon, 2003). Any defects in the visual field should be noted. One eye at a time should be tested, and the procedure should be repeated in each of the fields of gaze. If there is a field defect, the finger should be moved from the defective area to an area of better vision, and the location where the object is again visualized should be noted (Bickley).

Perimetry is also performed to ascertain a more accurate assessment of visual fields. Both kinetic and static perimetry approaches are used. When perimetry is conducted, the chin of the older adult must rest on a chin rest and one eye is covered as the patient looks at a central spot. Using a kinetic or static device, the patient is asked to signal when the stimulus is noticed. With kinetic perimetry, a moving stimulus is flashed to map the extent and sensitivity of the entire 360-degree field of vision. The Goldmann perimeter is often used for kinetic perimetry. With static perimetry, a nonmoving stimulus is flashed at different locations in the visual field. Stimuli are introduced with increasing levels of intensity until the stimulus is observed by the patient. Static perimetry is useful for evaluating the sensitivity of specific areas of the visual field, but is time consuming if used to map the entire visual field. The smaller the stimulus utilized when conducting perimetry, the greater the possibility of finding a scotoma (Pavan-Langston & Grosskreutz, 2002).

Extraocular Muscles

The corneal light reflex can be tested by asking the older adult to look straight ahead and shining a penlight on the bridge of the nose. The location of the corneal reflection in both eyes using a clock position as reference points should be noted. Normally the corneal reflex should be in the same position on each eye (Dillon, 2003). To check for conjugate eye movements, the patient should be asked to follow the examiner's finger through the six cardinal fields of gaze to reveal any abnormalities in movements of the eye muscles. Sometimes an older person may have difficulty focusing on near objects, so the examiner should make the distance the finger is held from the patient comfortable. If the older person moves his or her head instead of the eyes, assist the patient by holding the head in a midline position (Bickley, 2003). The extraocular eye muscles of each eye normally move together voluntarily in the same plane. Nystagmus should be noted. Nystagmus is a fine oscillation of the eyes, which is abnormal, except with an extreme left gaze. Normally the older adult should be able to follow the nurse's finger by moving eyes smoothly and symmetrically throughout the fields of gaze without moving the head (Dillon).

The cover/uncover test may also be helpful in assessing extraocular eye muscle alignment. Each eye should be covered and then uncovered when fixing the gaze straight ahead. The nurse should look for refixation of gaze with the uncovered eye. A steady gaze is normal. A refocusing means there is an asymmetry in the eye alignment. Generally glaucoma does not manifest with problems of extraocular eye muscles.

Pupils and Pupillary Reflex

Pupils normally should constrict with light and dilate during darkness. To observe the pupillary response, a beam of light should be directed at the pupil in a dark room. The procedure should be repeated in each eye. The consensual constriction in the opposite eye should be observed. The light should be directed toward the nasal aspect of the eye from the temporal area. The pupillary reflex assesses the integrity of the optic nerve. Neurological problems, such as increased intracranial pressure, head injury, tumor, cerebral vascular accident, hypoxia, or brain death, affect the pupillary light reflex. Certain medications may also have a negative effect (Dillon, 2003).

Anterior Chamber

The anterior chamber should be assessed as abnormalities may be found with infection or in response to trauma. The shadow test used to identify a shallow anterior chamber should be performed and may aid in glaucoma diagnosis. The older adult should look forward while the nurse shines a penlight at a 90-degree angle across the anterior chamber. With the penlight stationary, the light should be moved across the limbus of the eye toward the nose. A crescent-shaped shadow on the nasal side of the anterior chamber reflects a shallow anterior chamber that is characteristic of primary closed-angle glaucoma (Dillon, 2003).

External Structures

The external structures of the eye should be examined. Eyelashes should be present and curve outward and be free of drainage. Eyelids should cover one-half of the upper iris and have no crusting or lesions. The palpebral fissures should be symmetrical. There should be no protrusion of the eyeball beyond the frontal bone. The lacrimal gland and nasolacrimal duct should not have any edema, redness, or drainage. Conjunctiva should be smooth, pink, and clear with minimal visible blood vessels noted. Sclera should be smooth and white with the exception of some dark-skinned individuals who may have yellow or small brown spots on the sclera. The cornea is normally clear and smooth. In acute closed-angle glaucoma the cornea may be edematous. An edematous cornea occurs when excessive fluid passes into the cornea from the anterior chamber (Wilensky & Campbell, 2000). The iris should vary from green, blue, or brown and be circular. Pupils are round and equal. Small pupils are a result of injury to the pons, or may be the result of medications, such as narcotics or atropine. Central brain herniation occurs when the diencephalon shifts straight downward to the tentorium from an injury or a mass. When this occurs, the pupils become small and reactive and then fixed and dilated (Huether & McCance, 2004). Large, dilated pupils occur from using marijuana, mydriatic eye drops, anoxia, or cerebral herniation. Pupils dilate during cerebral herniation when the uncal or hippocampal gyrus shift from middle fossa to the posterior fossa of the brain as a result of an expanding cerebral mass (Huether & McCance, 2004). Unequal pupils may result from oculomotor damage, cerebral herniation, and increased intracranial pressure. The eyeballs should be gently palpated with the thumbs to assess for firmness. If the older adult has a known head injury or glaucoma, the eyeballs should not be palpated. Increased firmness of the eyeballs is characteristic of glaucoma.

Internal Structures

With an ophthalmoscope, the red reflex, optic disc, blood vessels, general retinal background, and macula should be observed. In glaucoma, it is especially important to note the size of the physiologic cup in the optic disc and compare it to the size of the optic disc. The cup should be half the size of the disc or less. The cup is white or lighter in comparison to the disc. With glaucoma there may be blurred optic disc margins. The arteries are smaller and brighter than the veins and have a light streak running through the middle of each one. The background normally is a yellow-orange-reddish color, but the pigment varies with the individual's skin pigment. The macula, the source of the sharpest vision, should be noted about two disc diameters on the temporal side of the optic disc margins.

Intraocular Pressure

The AAO (2000) recommends that only ophthalmologists measure IOP. IOP can be measured with a portable Tonopen. The Goldman applanation tonometer is the preferred instrument used in measuring IOP (AAO, 2003). The thickness of the central cornea, normally 540 to 555 μm, affects the IOP reading (AAO, 2002; Gordon et al., 2002). A thin central corneal thickness may produce a falsely low IOP reading. A thick central corneal thickness may produce a high IOP, even when the patient has normal vision and a normal optic disc (AAO, 2003). A thicker or thinner central corneal thickness is a risk factor in the detection of open-angle glaucoma in that it confuses the IOP measurement by applanation techniques (AAO, 2002; Gordon et al.).

REFERRAL TO AN OPHTHALMOLOGIST

The older adult should be referred to an ophthalmologist if any of the following findings are present: (a) a defect in the visual field suggestive of glaucoma, (b) the presence of optic nerve cupping, or (c) a suspected increase in IOP as noted by increased firmness of the eyeball on palpation. In addition to measuring IOP, the ophthalmologist will examine the older adult by using a slit-lamp to evaluate the anterior chamber, iris, lens, vitreous, eyelid margins, lashes, tear film, conjunctiva, sclera, and cornea (AAO, 2000a). Slit-lamp gonioscopy of the anesthetized cornea evaluates the cornea, central and peripheral anterior chamber depth, and any synechiae (AAO, 2000b; AAO, 2002). The ophthalmologist may measure corneal thickness if primary open-angle glaucoma is suspected (Gordon et al., 2002). To measure the corneal thickness (normal 0.50–0.65 mm), the ophthalmologist uses an electronic pachymeter attached to a slit-lamp (AAO, 2002). Wickham, Edmunds, and Murdoch (2003) recommend that measurements of central corneal thickness should be repeated because they can fluctuate over time.

MEDICAL MANAGEMENT

Medical management of the older adult with glaucoma primarily focuses on compliance with a multiple eye drop regime daily for the rest of the person's life. The patient may also take oral medications, such as acetazolamide. The absorption, metabolism, and excretion of medication in an older adult may be different from those in a younger person.

Refer to Tables 4.1 to 4.6 for commonly used medications in the treatment of angle-closure and open-angle glaucoma. Angle-closure glaucoma treatment includes miotics to flatten the peripheral iris and open the angle (Wilensky & Campbell, 2000) (Table 4.3). In addition, the severe pain of angle-closure glaucoma may require intramuscular morphine, or possibly a retrobulbar block. Miotics may also be used to treat open-angle glaucoma. Prostaglandin analogs (Table 4.4) may be used in the treatment of glaucoma to improve the outflow of aqueous humor. To decrease the production of aqueous humor, carbonic anhydrase inhibitors (Table 4.2), alpha$_2$-adrenergic agonists (Table 4.5), and beta-blockers (Table 4.1) may be used (Bartlett, Jaanus, Fiscella, & Sharir, 2001). Combination products are also available for the treatment of glaucoma (Table 4.6).

In addition to eye medications, the patient with glaucoma may need laser procedures or surgical interventions to improve drainage of the aqueous humor. There are several procedures that are used to treat glaucoma.

LASER PROCEDURES

Argon laser trabeculoplasty (ALT) is used to create holes in the trabecular meshwork to decrease outflow resistance. Laser (light amplification by stimulated emission of radiation) uses monochromatic light to beam a concentrated light in a small narrow focus. In ALT an intense focused light beam on a slit-lamp is used to cut or burn. It is most successful in patients over 65 year of age, with moderate to marked trabecular meshwork pigmentation, clear corneas, and primary open-angle glaucoma.

Laser iridectomy is indicated for acute angle-closure glaucoma (Aslanides & Katz, 2004). A laser iridectomy or a peripheral iridectomy may be performed prior to ALT to provide better visualization of the angle (Aslanides & Katz, 2004). Laser iridectomy is used as a diagnostic and a therapeutic modality with angle-closure glaucoma (Wilensky & Campbell, 2000). The procedure creates an opening in the iris and is indicated for acute and chronic angle-closure glaucoma associated with a pupillary block. In many cases, argon laser

TABLE 4.3 Miotics

Name/Dose	Action/Uses	Cautions/Side Effects	Nursing Concerns
		(Cholinergic Agonists/Parasympathomimetics/Cholinomimetics)	
Pilocarpine ocular system (Ocusert) (Pilocarpine 1%, 2%, or 4%) 1 drop 4 times a day or 1/2-inch gel ribbon once daily	Action: Acts directly on cholinergic receptors of the iris and ciliary body causing pupillary constriction, increased accommodation, and opening of the trabecular meshwork. Uses: primary open-angle glaucoma, acute management of angle-closure glaucoma	Ocular: stinging, accommodative spasm, miosis, cataracts, pupillary closure with angle-closure, retinal detachment, ciliary and conjunctival hyperemia, frontal headache, eye pain Systemic: rare—headache, brow ache, marked salivation, perspiration, bronchospasm, nausea, and vomiting; pulmonary edema, hypertension, hypotension, bradycardia, tachycardia, increased GI motility, respiratory paralysis Avoid if preexisting cataracts, under 40 years of age, history of retinal detachment and uncontrolled asthma.	Should be instituted gradually if myopia, aphakic, and with peripheral retinal disease

Source: Bartlett, J. D., Jaanus, S. D., Fiscella, R. G., & Sharir, M. (2001). Ocular hypotensive drugs. In J. D. Bartlett & S. D. Jaanus (Eds.), *Clinical ocular pharmacology* (4th ed., pp. 167–218). Boston, MA: Butterworth-Heinemann.

TABLE 4.4 Prostaglandin Analogs

Name/Dose	Action/Use	Caution/Side Effects	Nursing Concerns
Latanoprost (Xalatan) 0.005% 1 drop once daily in evening or bedtime	Action: Lowers IOP by increasing outflow Uses: 1st and 2nd line therapy for many types of glaucoma	Darkening of eyelid, increased iris pigmentation, conjunctival hyperemia, corneal erosion Systemic reactions—rare Contraindicated: history of uveitis, or prior ocular surgery	Additive therapy with other IOP reducing agents Well tolerated Refrigerate No cardiovascular or respiratory effects
Bimatoprost (Lumigan) 0.03% 1 drop once daily in evening	Action: Reduces IOP by increasing the outflow of aqueous humor through the trabecular meshwork.	Ocular: conjunctival hyperemia, growth of eyelashes, ocular pruritus, ocular burning, increased pigmentation of periocular skin and iris, tearing, blepharitis, photophobia Systemic: headache, hirsutism Contraindicated: hypersensitivity to bimatoprost, benzalkonium chloride, angle-closure glaucoma, Caution: in patients with renal or hepatic impairment, intraocular inflammation, or aphakia	
Uroprostone (Rescula) 0.12% 1 drop twice a day	Action: Enhances uveal scleral outflow. Uses: primary open-angle glaucoma and ocular hypertension, and normal-tension glaucoma	Contraindications: Same as Latanoprost Side effects: mild local eye disorders	

Source: American Society of Health-System Pharmacists. (2003). *AHFS drug handbook* (2nd ed.), Philadelphia, PA: Lippincott Williams, & Wilkins. Bartlett, J. D., Jaanus, S. D., Fiscella, R. G., & Sharir, M. (2001). Ocular hypotensive drugs. In J. D. Bartlett and S. D. Jaanus (Eds.), *Clinical ocular pharmacology* (4th ed., pp 167–218). Boston, MA: Butterworth-Heinemann.

TABLE 4.5 Alpha$_2$-Adrenergic Agonists

Name/Dose	Action/Use	Caution/Side Effects	Nursing Concerns
Apraclonidine (Iopidine) 0.5%, 1% 1 drop prior to or postprocedure	Action: decreased aqueous production Use: postsurgical elevations of IOP after laser trabeculectomy or iridotomy	Do not use with monoamine oxidase (MAO) inhibitors. Do not use if hypersensitive to clonidine. Ocular: Hypersensitivity effects include hyperemia, pruritus, discomfort, tearing, foreign body sensation.	Long-term use if limited by tachyphylaxis and allergic reactions
Brimonidine tartrate (Alphagan 0.2% with benzalkonium chloride) 1 drop twice a day or every 8 hours (Alphagan—P with pruite preservative) 0.15% 1 drop twice a day or every 8 hours	Action: Decrease aqueous production and increase the outflow through the trabecular meshwork.	Contraindicated with concomitant use of MAO inhibitors Caution in use with patients with Raynaud's phenenomen, orthostatic hypotension, or thromboangitis obliterans	When using the drug with benzalkonium chloride, insert soft lenses 15 minutes or more after administering Alphagan (to avoid soft lenses absorbing the Alphagan)

Sources: Facts and Comparisons. (2005). Agents for glaucoma. *Drug facts and comparisons 2006*. St. Louis, MO: Wolters Kluwer Health. Pavan-Langston, D., & Grosskreutz, C. (2002). Glaucoma. In D. Pavan-Langston (Ed.), *Manual of ocular diagnosis and therapy* (5th ed., pp. 251–285). Philadelphia: PA: Lippincott, Williams & Wilkins.

TABLE 4.6 Combination Agents

Name/Dose	Action/Use	Cautions/Side Effects	Nursing Concerns
Dorcolamide 2% Timolol maleate (Cosopt) 1 drop twice daily	Action as with dorzolamide and timolol Use: open-angle glaucoma	Ocular: burning, Systemic: abdominal pain, nausea, cough, dizziness, bradycardia	Combination product can be more convenient

Source: Bartlett, J. D., Jaanus, S., Fiscella, R. G., & Sharir, M. (2001). Ocular hypotensive drugs. In J. D. Bartlett and S. D. Jaanus (Eds.), *Clinical ocular pharmacology* (4th ed., pp. 167–218). Boston, MA: Butterworth-Heinemann.

iridectomy and laser iridectomy have replaced surgical iridectomy (Aslanides & Katz)

Prior to surgery, these patients receive IOP-lowering medications topically or orally. A lens is placed on the cornea, and laser energy is delivered through the cornea. Yttrium aluminum garnet (YAG) laser angle surgery may be used to treat open-angle glaucoma by tearing and dissolving the tissue (Pavan-Langston & Grosskreutz, 2002). Postoperatively steroids are used to reduce inflammation. The patient's preoperative eye medications are resumed after surgery.

Laser sclerostomy is another procedure that is performed internally with a probe or externally with a gonioscopy lens for patients who have excessive conjunctival scarring (Leen, 2004).

SURGICAL MANAGEMENT

A surgical trabeculectomy is the "gold standard" for glaucoma filtration surgery in treating uncontrolled POAG. A limbal fistula is created, which drains aqueous humor into the subconjunctival space. The procedure is also used to treat closed-angle glaucoma. Trabeculectomy is performed when medical therapy and laser procedures have failed. Trabeculectomy is also used if the patient has progressive glaucomatous cupping, visual field progression, excessive IOP, or if the patient is noncompliant or poorly tolerates medical therapy (Fellman, 2004).

Drainage implants, long tubes that drain aqueous from the anterior chamber to the episcleral plate, are used for refractory glaucoma when trabeculectomy surgery has failed (Freedman, 2004). Intraoperative complications are uncommon, but a tube misdirected into the anterior chamber, bleeding, and loss of anterior chamber can occur. Early postoperative complications include hypotony (low intraocular pressure), hemorrhagic effusions, and increased IOP. Late postoperative complications include elevation of IOP from a fibrous capsule (Freedman).

NURSE'S ROLE IN TREATMENT

By far, the most problematic aspect of care for the older adult with glaucoma is the need for medication compliance. Eye medications need to be consistently administered several times a day throughout the remainder of the older person's life. This can be particularly problematic because glaucoma, except for the acute episodes of closed-angle glaucoma, is a painless disease, which requires continued treatment regardless of the absence or presence of symptoms. For some, there may be a problem with motor skills needed for instilling eye drops, memory needed to remember to self-administer the medication, or cost of medication. Blindness from long-standing or inadequately treated glaucoma can often be prevented with proper timely diagnosis and treatment.

Nurses have a role in monitoring glaucoma treatment. Sheppard, Warner, and Kelley (2003) compared patients in a general physician-operated ophthalmic clinic to a nurse-led glaucoma-monitoring clinic on knowledge of symptoms, treatment, compliance with eye medications, and satisfaction. At 12-week follow-up, patients in the nurse-led glaucoma-monitoring clinic had fewer problems adhering to eye medications and were significantly more satisfied with treatment. There was no difference in knowledge of symptoms, compliance with eye medications, or treatment.

The proper administration of eye medications should be adhered to by the nurse and taught to the older adult and family members if the patient is unable to provide self-care. Hands should always be washed before administering eye drops. The patient should look up, and the lower lid should be gently retracted to expose the conjunctiva. Without touching the conjunctival surface with the medication bottle, 1 drop of medication should be instilled. Excess should be wiped with a tissue. Multiple eye drops should be spaced 5 minutes apart. The lid of the dropper should be placed on its side to prevent contamination. The patient should be taught how to do lacrimal occlusion (AAO, 2002). After administering the eye drops, the inner canthus should be lightly pressed against the bone for several seconds. This occludes the puncta of the lacrimal gland, thereby minimizing the systemic absorption of the eye drops.

The nurse's role in the surgical treatment of glaucoma is also important. The nursing care of the patient undergoing a trabeculoplasty includes eye drops to decrease IOP, visual acuity checks, and monitoring vital signs before and after laser surgery. Discharge teaching should include medication administration, safety, and follow-up with the physician. The older adult should be advised to call the physician for any increased symptoms following surgery such as headache pain or nausea.

The nurse who participates in care of patients with glaucoma has an opportunity to help preserve sight of patients. Glaucoma is often not the primary reason for hospital admission. When the older adult is admitted to the hospital for another problem, preexisting glaucoma should alert the nurse to possible limitations in self-care and the need for continued treatment with eye medications and monitoring of the progression of the disease.

Preserving independence at home is of primary importance to the older adult. Because glaucoma is a lifelong problem, there are many opportunities for patient teaching. There are also many community resources for the visually impaired that provide support and assistance to the older adult with glaucoma and family members. Low-tech assistive devices such as magnifying glasses, as well as advanced and expensive technological devices such as computers for the blind, are available. For the older person, vision rehabilitation specialists can assist patients to maximize remaining abilities with modifications at home. Social workers can assist in finding financial resources for the visually impaired. A collaborative approach to the management of glaucoma, which may be initiated by the nurse, will promote a higher quality of life for the older adult.

REFERENCES

American Academy of Ophthalmology. (2000a). *Preferred practice patterns—Comprehensive adult medical eye evaluation.* San Francisco, CA: *American Academy of Ophthalmology,* 1–17. Retrieved on July 1, 2004, from http://www/aao/org.

American Academy of Ophthalmology. (2000b). *Preferred practice patterns—Primary angle closure.* San Francisco, CA: *American Academy of Ophthalmology,* 1–21. Retrieved July 1, 2004, from http://www.aao.org.

American Academy of Ophthalmology. (2002). *Preferred practice patterns—Primary open angle glaucoma suspect, limited revision.* San Francisco, CA: *American Academy of Ophthalmology,* 1–27. Retrieved on July 1, 2004, from http:// www. aao.org.

American Academy of Ophthalmology. (2003). *Preferred practice patterns—Primary Open-angle glaucoma, limited revision.* San Francisco, CA: *American Academy of Ophthalmology,* 1–37. Retrieved on July 1, 2004, from http://www.aao.org.

American Society of Health-System Pharmacists. (2003). *AHFS drug handbook* (2nd ed.). Philadelphia: PA: Lippincott Williams & Wilkins.

Aslanides, I. M., & Katz, L. J. (2004). Argon laser trabeculoplasty and peripheral iridectomy. In M. Yanoff & J. S. Duker (Eds.), *Ophthalmology* (2nd ed., pp. 1557–1561). St. Louis, MO: Mosby.

Bartlett, J. D., Jaanus, S. D., Fiscella, R. G., & Sharir, M. (2001). Ocular hypotensive drugs. In J. D. Bartlett & S. D. Jaanus (Eds.), *Clinical ocular pharmacology* (4th ed., pp. 167–218). Boston, MA: Butterworth Heinemann.

Bickley, L. S. (2003). *Bates' guide to physical examination and history taking* (8th ed.) Philadelphia, PA: Lippincott Williams & Wilkins.

Desai, M., Pratt, L., Lentzner, H., & Robinson, K. (2001). *Trends in vision and hearing among older Americans: Aging trend, No. 2.* Hyattsville, MD: National Centers for Health Statistics.

Dillon, P. (2003). *Nursing health assessment. A critical thinking, case studies approach.* Philadelphia, PA: F. A. Davis Co.

Distelhorst, J. S., & Hughes, G. M. (2003). Open angle glaucoma. *American Family Physician, 67*(9), 1937–1945.

Facts and Comparisons. (2005). Agents for glaucoma. *Drug facts and comparisons 2006.* St. Louis, MO: Wolters Kluwer Health.

Fellman, R. (2004). Trabeculectomy. In M. Yanoff & J. S. Duker (Eds.), *Ophthalmology* (2nd ed., pp. 1586–1599). St. Louis, MO: Mosby.

Freedman, J. (2004). Drainage implants. In M. Yanoff & J. S. Duker (Eds.), *Ophthalmology* (2nd ed., pp. 1604–1609). St. Louis, MO: Mosby.

Gordon, M. O., Beiser, J. A., Brandt, J. D., Heuier, D. K., Higginbotham, E. J., Johnson, et al. (2002). The ocular hypertension treatment study: Baseline factors that predict the onset of primary open-angle glaucoma. *Archives of Ophthalmology, 120,* 714–720.

Huether, S. E., & McCance, K. L. (2004). *Understanding pathophysiology* (3rd ed.). St. Louis, MO: Mosby.

Kappes, J., & McNair, R. (2003). Headache and visual changes at triage: Do not allow the patient's assumptions to cloud your critical thinking. *Journal of Emergency Nursing, 29*(6), 584–594.

Lacy, C. F., Armstrong, L. L., Goldman, M. P., & Lance, L. L. (2005). *Lexi-Comp's drug information handbook* (13th ed.). Hudson, OH: Lexi-Comp.

Leen, M. M. (2004). Laser filtration procedures. In M. Yanoff & J. S. Duker (Eds.), *Ophthalmology* (2nd ed., pp. 1562—1564). St. Louis, MO: Mosby.

Pavan-Langston, D., & Grosskreutz, C. (2002). Glaucoma. In D. Pavan-Langston (Ed.), *Manual of ocular diagnosis and therapy* (5th ed., pp. 251–285). Philadelphia, PA: Lippincott, Williams & Wilkins.

Sheppard, J., Warner, J., & Kelley, L. (2003). An evaluation of the effectiveness of a nurse-led glaucoma monitoring clinic. *Ophthalmic nursing: International Journal of Ophthalmic Nursing, 7*(2), 15–21.

Wickham, L., Edmunds, B., & Murdoch, I. (2003). Central corneal thickness: Will one measurement suffice? *Ophthalmology, 112,* 225–228.

Wilensky, J. T., & Campbell, D. G. (2000). Primary angle-closure glaucoma. In F. A. Jakobiec, D. T. Azar, & E. Gragoudas (Eds.), *Principles and practice of ophthalmology* (2nd ed., Vol. 4, pp. 2685–2705). Philadelphia, PA: Saunders.

CHAPTER 5

Retinopathies

Judith M. Pentedemos

Retinopathy is a noninflammatory disorder of the retina that may occur in older adults. It may be present without symptomatology, and therefore the health care provider is urged to screen for it during the physical examination. Although often asymptomatic, its presence is always sequela to another process. The most common causes for the development of retinopathy in the older adult are type 1 diabetes mellitus (DM), type 2 DM, and hypertension (HTN). Other conditions responsible for the development of retinopathy are autoimmune disorders, anemia, sickle cell disease, trauma, and the retinopathy of prematurity. This chapter focuses on the most common types of retinopathy in the older adult: diabetic and hypertensive.

Just as type 2 DM and HTN can have insidious onsets, so do the retinopathies associated with them. This can present a particular challenge for the health care provider, who all too often discovers the retinopathy before the causative disorder. Thus, all health care providers are encouraged to become skilled in performing an ophthalmoscopic examination as part of every annual physical examination of the older adult for the purpose of early detection.

Early detection of retinopathy should result in early referral to an ophthalmologist for an in-depth ophthalmoscopic examination. Depending on findings, further diagnostics or interventions may be necessary to control the condition.

EPIDEMIOLOGY

Diabetic Retinopathy

The National Health and Nutrition Examination Survey (NHANES) is the only nationally representative survey that examined the prevalence of diagnosed and undiagnosed DM and impaired fasting glucose (IFG) in the U.S. population from 1999 to 2000 (Morbidity and Mortality Weekly Report [MMWR], 2003). The prevalence of DM and IFG in adults ($\geq$20 years old) was estimated to be 29 million. Of this figure, 16.7 million adults had diagnosed and undiagnosed type 1 and type 2 DM, and 12.3 million had IFG (MMWR). Without intervention, those with IFG will develop type 2 DM. By the year 2025, diabetes rates are expected to double (Wilkinson, 2003). This projected increase is due to the anticipated higher numbers of Americans over the age of 65 and the increase in obesity rates, resulting in an increase in the incidences of IFG and type 2 DM (Ciulla, Amador, & Zinman, 2003). An increase in the incidence of complications from diabetes, such as diabetic retinopathy, will be an unfortunate consequence of this epidemic.

Currently, diabetic retinopathy is the third most common cause of blindness in the United States and the leading cause of new blindness in adults ages 20 to 74. It is responsible for about 24,000 new cases of blindness yearly (Brown, Pedula, & Summers, 2003). The onset of diabetic retinopathy differs between type 1 DM and type 2 DM. An individual with type 1 DM rarely develops vision-threatening retinopathy in the first 3 to 5 years after diagnosis or before puberty. However, after 20 years with type 1 DM, most adults will have developed it to some degree. Unlike type 1 DM, up to 21% of individuals with type 2 DM already have retinopathy at the time that their diabetes is diagnosed, and most will develop it over time (Fong et al., 2004).

Descriptions of diabetic retinopathy began to appear in the literature between 1930 and 1940 (Pfeifer, 1998). For years, health care providers thought that no matter what was done for treatment of diabetes, complications from diabetes were inevitable (Beaser, 2001). It was not known if retinopathy was a condition associated directly with the diabetes or the result of poor blood sugar control (Pfeifer). Subsequently, several studies were performed for the purpose of identifying the relationship between improved blood sugar control and the incidence of diabetic complications, such as the development and progression of retinopathy. These landmark studies, the Diabetes Control and Complications Trial (DCCT), the U.K. Prospective Diabetes Study (UKPDS), the Kumamoto Study, the Wisconsin Epidemiologic Study of Diabetic Retinopathy (WESDR), and others collectively confirmed for health care providers that control of hyperglycemia and HTN could prevent retinopathy (Brown et al., 2003). As a result of these findings, health care providers adopted a preventative or proactive approach to the management of DM for the purposes of health maintenance and prevention of co-morbidities (Beaser).

Hypertensive Retinopathy

Most health care providers readily accept claims that prevention of cardiovascular disease involves controlling multiple risk factors through healthy diet, weight reduction, regular physical exercise, and management of blood pressure (BP) elevations. NHANES provided the earliest data on the success of these interventions between 1976 and 1991. NHANES demonstrated that there was an increased awareness and improved treatment and control of HTN, which seemed to contribute to reductions in cardiovascular morbidity and mortality (Fodera, 2003). NHANES III (1991–1994) data reported declining trends in BP management with only 27% of the hypertensive Americans being managed appropriately with a BP less than 140/90 mm Hg. NHANES data more recently reflect 35% of adults with HTN being adequately managed (Fodera).

In May 2003, The National Heart Lung and Blood Institute (NHLBI) released the Joint National Committee on Prevention, Detection, Evaluation, and Treatment of High Blood Pressure (JNC 7). The JNC 7 described categories, diagnostic criteria, and treatment recommendations for normal BP, prehypertension, and HTN (Stages 1 and 2). The report also issued recommendations for more stringent management of BP in individuals with DM as well as for proper BP measurement guidelines for standardization.

The prevalence of HTN among Americans is estimated to be 58 million (Lewis, 2003). Although the incidence of HTN increases with age, treatment rates do not increase. In a sample of 5,192 patients, treatment for HTN differed significantly among three age groups: under age 60, 60 to 79 years old, and 80 years and older (Lewis, 2004). Overall, 66% of individuals were treated with antihypertensive agent(s). However, among patients age 80 and older, there was not a significant increase in treatment despite the fact that there was a significant increase in HTN (Lewis).

The American Diabetes Association (ADA, 2005) informs that there are no long-term studies demonstrating the benefits of tight glycemic, lipid, or hypertensive control in persons over 65 years of age, although there is much evidence that there is a high prevalence of DM and HTN among older adults. The incidence of DM and HTN is also more prevalent among certain ethnic groups: African Americans, Hispanic Americans, Native Americans, Asian Americans, and Pacific Islanders. Health care providers should be aware of the conditions inherent to their client population and screen for them on a regular basis.

ANATOMY

The retina, analogous to the film in a camera, is a multilevel structure, each level having a different function and composition. Light entering the eye must pass through the transparent anterior retinal layers to reach the photoreceptors and retinal pigment epithelium. The photoreceptors (rods and cones) convert the light energy to nerve impulses that are transmitted through the nerve fiber layer to the optic nerve and then to the brain for interpretation. The vascular supply of the retina consists of the retinal blood vessels that supply the inner half of the retina and the choroidal vasculature, which serves the outer half. These vessels supply the oxygen and nutrients needed to keep the structures viable.

The conditions of hypertensive and diabetic retinopathy occur as a result of DM and HTN causing changes to the retinal microvasculature. The factors that influence the onset and progression of retinopathy are particular to each condition. An individual with one condition may develop the other condition, and aggressive treatment of both conditions may be necessary to minimize vision loss.

DIABETIC RETINOPATHY

Pathophysiology of Diabetic Retinopathy

Diabetic retinopathy is classified as a microvascular disease and a co-morbid condition of both type 1 and type 2 DM. The incidence increases in direct relationship to the duration of DM. Retinopathy occurs when the small blood vessels nourishing the retina become damaged. Clinical evidence suggests that diabetic retinopathy occurs as a consequence of the metabolic derangements of hyperglycemia. Several metabolic events, all driven by hyperglycemia, appear to be involved in the development of this condition.

An early process of nonenzymatic glycosylation refers to the method by which glucose chemically attaches to the amino group of proteins without the aid of enzymes. These early attachments with proteins are chemically reversible and do not result in further damage. The degree of enzymatic glycosylation is directly related to the level of blood glucose. Hence, the measurement of glycosylated hemoglobin or hemoglobin A_{1c} (HbA$_{1c}$ or A_{1c}) is a useful indicator of the effectiveness of diabetes management. When not reversed by a reduction in blood glucose, the early products of glycosylation undergo a slow series of chemical rearrangements to form irreversible advanced glycosylation end products (AGE). The end products have a number of chemical and biologic properties that adhere to and destroy the blood vessel walls.

In capillaries, plasma proteins such as albumin bind to the glycosylated basement membrane, resulting in increased membrane thickening that leads to structural and functional defects. AGEs bind to receptors on endothelium and leukocytes and incite monocyte emigration, release of cytokines and growth factors from macrophages, increased endothelial permeability, increased pro-coagulant activity on endothelial cells and macrophages, and enhanced proliferation of and synthesis of extracellular matrix by fibroblasts and smooth muscle cells. All of these activities combine to result in the microvascular disease of diabetic retinopathy.

Along with the aforementioned extracellular hyperglycemic changes, intracellular hyperglycemia causes disruption in some tissues that do not require insulin for glucose transport, such as nerves, kidneys, blood vessels, and lenses. Hyperglycemia leads to an increase in intracellular glucose that is then metabolized via the polyol pathway by the enzyme aldose reductase to sorbitol, a polyol, and eventually to fructose. The accumulated levels of sorbitol and fructose lead to increased intracellular osmolarity, with an influx of water, and osmotic cell injury. In the lens, the water causes swelling and opacity, which can cause vision changes. In the vasculature of the eye, the sorbitol is absorbed by pericytes. The pericyte cells (supportive cells of the retinal vasculature) become damaged, and blood components are allowed to leak through the blood vessel walls leading to microaneurysms, hard exudates of albumin, microischemia, and microinfarctions. Other sequelae include abnormal permeability, capillary nonperfusion, and neovascularization (Crawford & Cotran, 1999).

Assessing for Diabetic Retinopathy

As the majority of older adults with retinopathy from diabetes or HTN are asymptomatic, the health care provider must devise a method to routinely assess the client for the condition. This should be done at least annually via a review of systems (ROS) and by ophthalmoloscopic examination.

The first step to evaluation of vision is the ROS. During the ROS, information should be elicited about episodes of visual changes between visits, including blurring, vision loss, floaters or increased number of floaters, or flashes of light, as these may be symptoms of diabetic retinopathy. Inquiry as to the date of the last examination with the optometrist or ophthalmologist, what the findings were, and whether a dilated eye examination was performed is important.

Due to the physiologic changes that take place in the eye during hyperglycemic episodes, patients who formerly could see clearly at a distance rather suddenly find that they are myopic, and patients who had required reading glasses (bifocals) find that they can read better without them. Although distance vision has decreased, patients often consider the increase in near vision as an improvement in sight. Individuals with diabetes often state that their vision is better or worse at certain times of the day and there may be evidence of refractive changes. This may be indicative of hyperglycemia and should be corrected before the individual is prescribed corrective lenses. Other visual complaints can be indicative of hypoglycemia. These are not refractive errors,

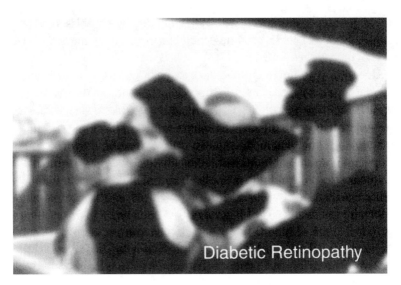

FIGURE 5.1 Seen by individual with diabetic retinopathy.
Source: National Eye Institute, National Institutes of Health.

but are due to the effects of hypoglycemia on the central nervous system. Commonly patients report that a pattern or aura precedes these episodes. They may report a brightening of the surroundings, flashes, sparks of lights, dark spots, darkening, or narrowing vision.

After the ROS, visual acuity should be examined with each eye tested independently, preferably with glasses on. The patient may be observed shifting his or her head instinctively for better visualization. This may be a sign that the patient is suffering from low vision, as there may be a part of their visual field lost to retinopathy (Figure 5.1).

The next step toward diagnosis of retinopathy is the ophthalmoscopic examination. This should take place in a darkened room. In general primary health care settings, the typical eye exam is done without dilating the pupils. It is limited and prevents a thorough examination of the posterior retinal surface. To dilate the pupil, mydriatic eye drops may be instilled, if there are no contraindications (narrow-angle glaucoma). Dilation allows for viewing of the peripheral retina and evaluation of the macular area. An ophthalmic exam with dilation allows for better investigation of unexplained visual loss. By using a nonmydriatic ophthalmoscope (PanOptic) that allows viewing of the retina that is three to five times wider than that of a standard direct ophthalmoscope, there is an increased likelihood that retinopathy will be identified in the general practice setting (Gill, Cole, Lebowitz, & Diamond, 2004).

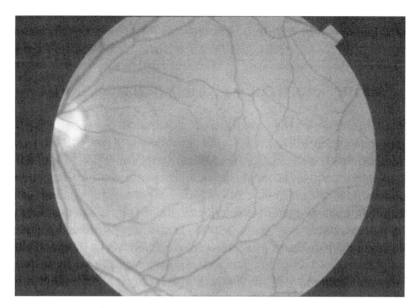

FIGURE 5.2 Normal retina.
Source: National Eye Institute, National Institutes of Health.

Most health assessment textbooks provide detailed instructions on how to perform an ophthalmologic exam. The best advice to becoming proficient at performing this exam is to practice the skill. Looking at photographs of healthy retinas (Figure 5.2) and diseased retinas (Figure 5.3) to become familiar with the structures, landmarks, and colorings is helpful in increasing proficiency in ophthalmic exams. This type of preparation is beneficial prior to the performance of the ophthalmic examinations. Due to structural changes in the older adult, pupils are typically smaller and more sluggish, and it is very difficult for older adults to tolerate the bright light of the ophthalmoscope. A mentor, such as an ophthalmologist or optometrist who can assist with technique and give advice for successful examinations and documentation, is also helpful to assist in perfecting ophthalmologic assessment skills. Findings should be documented and diagrammed for future reference.

Classification of Diabetic Retinopathy

Typically, DR progresses through stages, from mild nonproliferative to proliferative, with characteristic findings specific to each stage (Table 5.1). Currently, the vast majority of health care providers do not use a standardized set of definitions to describe the severity of DR even though classification schemes exist (Wilkinson, 2003). It is important that the terminology be standardized to

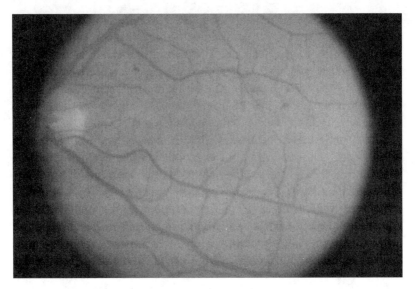

FIGURE 5.3 Nonproliferative diabetic retinopathy.
Source: National Eye Institute, National Institutes of Health.

allow health care providers to recognize that the levels of DR dictate the degree of urgency for referral. In a workshop held in April 2002, the International Congress of Ophthalmology proposed a clinical disease severity scale for the purpose of universal terminology and disease classification (Wilkinson). No apparent DR, the first stage in the proposed scale, identifies individuals with diabetes who have no clinical evidence of retinopathy. The workshop participants identified this as an important distinction as the incidence of progression to sight-threatening proliferative retinopathy is greater if the individual has microaneurysms or hemorrhages at the time of diagnosis (Wilkinson).

Nonproliferative DR

Nonproliferative DR is divided into three distinct stages: mild, moderate, and severe. In mild nonproliferative DR, microaneurysms, which are the result of capillary basement membrane changes resulting in an out-pouching of the vessel wall and eventual capillary rupture, are the only findings. The microaneurysm, when filled with blood, appears as a tiny red dot with discrete borders. This stage is not associated with a significant risk of imminent proliferative disease and requires only periodic reevaluation.

When the microaneurysms are surrounded by a ring of serous fluid (soft exudates), or yellow lipid (hard exudates), the degree of retinopathy has

TABLE 5.1 DR: Levels, Subjective and Objective Data

Level of Disease Severity	Subjective Data	Objective Data*
No apparent DR	None	No abnormalities
Mild nonproliferative DR	Generally none	Microaneurysms only
Moderate nonproliferative DR	Usually none	Microaneurysms and venous anomalies, soft exudates (cotton wool spots), hard exudates, dot/blot hemorrhages,
Severe nonproliferative DR	Frequently none, floaters, reduced vision	Above findings and any of the following: 20 or more intraretinal hemorrhages in 4 quadrants; venous beading in 2 or more quadrants; intraretinal micro-vascular abnormalities in 1 or more quadrants w/o neovascularization
Proliferative DR	Occasionally none, floaters, reduced vision, blurred vision	Above findings and 1 or more of the following: neovascularization preretinal or vitreous hemorrhage

*Findings observable with dilated ophthalmologic exam.
Source: Adapted with permission from Beaser, R. S. (2001). Microvascular complications. In R. S. Beaser & the staff of Joslin Diabetes Center (Eds.), *Joslin's diabetes deskbook: A guide for primary care providers* (pp. 373–396). Boston, MA: Joslin Diabetes Center; and Wilkinson, C. P. (2003, September 8). *Classification of diabetic retinopathy: A proposed international clinical disease severity grading scale for diabetic retinopathy and diabetic macular edema.* Retrieved November 25, 2003, from http://www.medscape.com/viewprogram/2600_pnt.
Copyright 2003 by Joslin Diabetes Center, Boston, MA. All rights reserved. Adapted with permission.

progressed to moderate nonproliferative. Exudates are the result of vascular leakage, but the specific leaking of the microaneurysm may not be visible ophthalmoscopically. Intraretinal hemorrhages that occur with DR are described either as red dots or blots or as flame-shaped hemorrhages.

Nonproliferative retinopathy may also include abnormalities, such as superficial white lesions with feathery edges known as cotton-wool spots. The cotton-wool spots are indicative of progressive ischemia, caused by microvascular obstructions and nonperfusion of the capillaries due to thrombus formation within the microaneurysm, resulting in infarction of the nerve fiber layer of the retina. Eventually more ominous ischemic lesions occur. These include irregular dilations of retinal veins, called venous beading, intraretinal microvascular abnormalities, and extensive retinal hemorrhages.

The classification of severe nonproliferative DR is established when any of the following are observed: 20 or more intraretinal hemorrhages in four quadrants, definite venous beading in two or more quadrants, or prominent

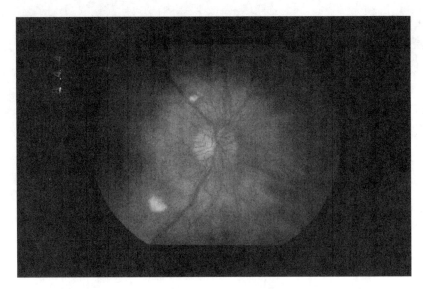

FIGURE 5.4 Proliferative retinopathy.
Source: National Eye Institute, National Institutes of Health.

intraretinal microvascular abnormalities (IRMA) occur in one or more quadrants. There is no evidence of new vessels (neovascularization) growing at this stage (Wilkinson, 2003). The level of nonproliferative DR establishes the risk of progression to sight-threatening proliferative retinopathy and helps one to establish the appropriate clinical management (Beaser, 2001).

Proliferative DR

Proliferative retinopathy (Figure 5.4) is the last and most ominous stage of DR as it is responsible for severe vision loss. The vision loss is due to new vessels growing on the optic disc (NVD) or new vessels growing elsewhere on the retina (NVE). NVD and NVE are the result of retinal ischemia that has occurred as a consequence of thrombus formation, capillary destruction, and hemorrhage. The delicate new vessels resemble a tangle of hair or a fishnet. They are especially fragile and rupture easily, causing preretinal hemorrhage or vitreous hemorrhage within the eye. Vitreous hemorrhages may be mild and perceived by the individual as dark spots or floaters. However, they may be severe and fill the vitreous compartment with blood, decreasing the patient's visual acuity to light perception only. A vitreous hemorrhage is an ophthalmic emergency, and individuals with these symptoms should be examined immediately by an ophthalmologist to rule out other potential causes of a vitreous hemorrhage, such as retinal detachment. The new vessels may be accompanied by the growth of fibrous tissue, which may cause traction or pulling on the retina, resulting in traction retinal detachment.

Once retinopathy has been identified in the general practice setting, the older adult should be referred to a qualified optometrist or ophthalmologist for an in-depth ophthalmoscopic exam. Individuals with type 2 DM should have annual ophthalmoscopic examinations starting with diagnosis, and those with type 1 DM, whether young or old, should be evaluated within 3 to 5 years of diagnosis and annually thereafter (American Diabetes Association, 2005).

Macular Edema

Although retinopathies are the focus of this chapter, the potential for the development of diabetic macular edema (DME) should be mentioned. DME is caused by fluid leaking from retinal vessels and accumulating in the macula. It can be present with either nonproliferative or proliferative diabetic retinopathy. DME is difficult to detect with a regular ophthalmologic exam (Beaser, 2001). It is defined as retinal thickening and may range in severity from mild DME to severe DME. Determining the severity of DME requires a three-dimensional assessment that is best performed through a dilated pupil using a slip-lamp with accessory lenses and/or stereo fundus photography (Wilkinson, 2003). An individual with DME may not experience any symptoms; however, a mild blurring of central vision frequently occurs. Distortion of straight lines may also be present (Beaser, 2001; Wilkinson, 2003).

HYPERTENSIVE RETINOPATHY

Pathophysiology of Hypertensive Retinopathy

Like diabetic retinopathy, hypertensive retinopathy (HR) results from changes to the retinal microvasculature. In hypertensive retinopathy, the increased pressure placed on the tunica intima of the medium and large arteries leads to arteriosclerotic plaque formation and eventual reduction in the lumen size of these vessels. This allows superficial hemorrhages and microinfarcts (cotton-wool spots) to develop. In extreme cases, disc edema develops. A HTN-related increase in intracranial pressure may cause this phenomenon, which produces papilledema. The exact mechanism is poorly understood. The cotton-wool spots develop in 24 to 48 hours when the diastolic BP is ≥110 mm Hg and can resolve in 2 to 10 weeks once the BP is controlled. The arteriosclerotic changes persist even when systemic blood pressure is normalized. A ring of lipid exudates that remain in the retina after leakage occurs from fragile capillaries may form what is referred to as a macular star. The macular star develops within a few weeks of the elevated BP and resolves within months to years after the BP is reduced. Papilledema may develop within days to weeks of increased BP and resolves within weeks to months after the BP is lowered (Sowka, Gurwood, & Kabat, 2001).

Assessing for Hypertensive Retinopathy

Assessment of the older adult for HR includes a health history, ROS, examination of the individual's visual acuity, assessment of BP, and ophthalmoscopic exam. The health history should assess the older adult's diet, exercise and activity level, as well as past and present alcohol and tobacco use, as these are risk factors for vascular diseases such as HTN and atherosclerosis. The ROS may be positive for headaches and vague visual disturbances in the older adult with hypertensive retinopathy. It is crucial to accurately and properly assess the BP. To properly assess the BP, the individual should be allowed to sit quietly for 5 minutes in a chair with feet on the floor, as climbing onto an examination table and sitting without back support can be physically challenging to the older adult resulting in an abnormally elevated BP. The bladder of the BP cuff should cover 80% of the arm circumference and should be applied above the anticubital fossa. The individual's arm should be supported at the level of his or her heart during the procedure.

The ophthalmoscopic exam of older adults who have HR reveals cotton-wool spots and flame-shaped hemorrhages. Only rarely will there be retinal or macular edema. A macular star is not common but may form in the area from the disc to the macula in advanced stages, and papilledema will be present in the latest stage (Sowka et al., 2001). A narrowing of the blood vessels is evidence of hypertensive changes in the arterioles. In acute HTN and with the onset of malignant HTN, these changes initially appear as focal spasms in the vessels. In chronic HTN, the narrowing is more diffuse. The arteriolar walls appear thickened, almost hyaline (silvery) or onion-skinned (Albert and Dryja, 1999). Arteriosclerosis is often found concurrently and is evidenced by arteriolar narrowing, arteriovenous crossing changes with venous constriction, arteriolar color changes, and vessel sclerosis (Sowka et al.). HR is categorized as follows:

- Grade I: Generalized narrowing of the arterioles
- Grade II: Grade I changes and focal arteriolar spasms
- Grade III: Grade II changes, flame-shaped hemorrhages, dot-blot hemorrhages, cotton-wool spots, and hard waxy exudates
- Grade IV: All Grade III changes plus papilledema (Albert & Dryja).

It should be pointed out that hypertensive retinopathy presents with a "dry" retina, that is, few hemorrhages, rare edema, rare exudates, and multiple cotton-wool spots; whereas diabetic retinopathy presents with a "wet" retina from multiple hemorrhages, multiple exudates, extensive edema, and few cotton-wool spots. A diastolic BP of at least 110 mm Hg is needed for cotton-wool spots to develop from HTN. Malignant HTN, typically in the range of 250/150 mm Hg, is required for papilledema to develop. With the presence of malignant hypertension, the patient should be transported to a hospital emergency room for admission and treatment, as this should be considered a medical crisis (Sowka et al., 2001).

DIAGNOSTIC TESTING FOR RETINOPATHIES

Referral to an ophthalmologist is necessary whenever a retinopathy is suspected or identified, as an ophthalmologist has the ability to take photographs of the fundus and to perform a fluorescein angiogram for the purpose of diagnosis and treatment. Proper fundus photographs require a photographer skilled in obtaining photographs and a reader skilled in the interpretation of the photographs. Recent techniques and digital technology allow high-quality photographs to be taken through undilated pupils. This technology may eventually permit undilated photographic retinopathy screening both in the office as well as via telemedicine (Barclay, 2002).

A fluorescein scan (angiogram) can be done in the ophthalmologist's office to identify areas of vascular leakage, nonperfusion, and neovascularization. Fluorescein, a yellow dye that fluoresces under cobalt-blue light, enhances visibility of the microvascular structures of the retina and choroid. The procedure begins with dilation of the pupil, unless contraindicated. Once the pupils are sufficiently dilated, fluorescein is injected rapidly into the anticubital vein. The fluorescein reaches the retina in approximately 12 to 15 seconds. The choridal vessels and choriocapillaries fill with fluorescein, illuminating the retina for what is known as the choroidal flush. The dye continues into the arteries, capillaries, and veins. Approximately 30 to 60 minutes after the injection, the fluorescein is hardly visible in the retinal vessels. Photographs, taken in succession from beginning to end, are interpreted by the ophthalmologist.

In cases of HR, there is no indication to perform fluorescein angiography, as it yields no diagnostic information (Sowka et al., 2001).

MANAGEMENT OF RETINOPATHIES

The treatment of diabetic or HR in the older adult is addressed by managing the underlying disease according to acceptable standards or clinical guidelines. These guidelines include screening for the condition, diagnostic criteria, management options ranging from diet and exercise to medication, follow-up/reevaluation schedules, and recommendations for referral to a specialist.

Diabetes Management

The ADA (2005) published the revised Standards of Medical Care in Diabetes, which are important guidelines in the care of older adults with diabetes. The ADA recommends that individuals with DM receive medical care from a physician-coordinated team. The team may include physicians, nurse practitioners, physician's assistants, nurses, dietitians, pharmacists, mental health professionals, family members, and the patient. A collaborative team approach with individualized patient goals and emphasis on empowerment through education should be most beneficial to the older adult with DM.

Management should include educating the older adult in the self-monitoring of blood glucose (SMBG). This empowers the individual to control blood glucose through self-awareness of the factors that influence blood sugar (ADA, 2005). Individuals should be encouraged to record their blood sugars on a graph and to document what they perceive to be the causes of any abnormal blood sugar level. The data will prove to be an invaluable learning tool and may help to modify behaviors. The blood glucose monitor is likened to a camera, recording one moment in time, whereas the A_{1c} is the motion picture capturing every moment. The A_{1c} (glycosylated hemoglobin, glycohemoglobin, hemoglobin A_{1c}) is the gold standard of diabetes management. The A_{1c} is an *average* of an individual's blood sugar during the 90 days prior to the test. As it is an average, the health care provider should interpret it in conjunction with the blood sugars reported by the patient, as multiple low blood sugar reactions in conjunction with elevated blood sugars can reduce an A_{1c} to an acceptable level. The A_{1c} alone does not reflect the patterns of blood sugar management that allow the health care provider to adjust medications. With control of blood sugar close to normoglycemia, there has been an associated reduction in microvascular complications of DM (ADA).

Although it is important to control blood sugar to near normoglycemia, it is important to note that sudden improvement in blood sugar control, often seen when starting multiple daily injections or insulin pump therapy, can lead to a transient worsening of retinopathy. This should not deter the health care provider from initiating tight control. The health care provider should anticipate this occurrence and refer individuals for a dilated retinal evaluation prior to initiating intensive insulin therapy or aggressive oral therapy (Beaser, 2001).

Although blood sugar is one factor in diabetes management, there are several others. Lipid management should be aimed at lowering LDL cholesterol (<100 mg/dl), raising HDL cholesterol (>40 mg/dl), and lowering triglycerides (<150 mg/dl). Although the benefits of lipid management are related to the prevention of macrovascular complications, the promotion of weight loss and control of HTN are also important to minimize atherosclerotic plaque formation. HTN should be controlled to <130/80 mm Hg, and it is recommended that those individuals with DM be prescribed an angiotensin-converting enzyme (ACE) inhibitor (ADA, 2005; Joint National Committee, NHLBI, 2004). If an older adult is unable to tolerate ACE inhibitor therapy, an angiotensin II receptor blocker (A2RB) may be substituted (ADA).

When caring for the older adult with DM, the health care provider should be aware that anemia can lead to the development of DR, with progressive proliferative DR having been reported within 6 to 12 months after the anemia was diagnosed (Bridge & Hirsch, 2001). The condition of anemia reduces the oxygen-carrying capacity of the red blood cells, resulting in tissue hypoxia. In addition, tissue hypoxia develops as the result of the products of glycosylation. High blood sugar causes an elevation in glycosylated hemoglobin levels, and glycosylated hemoglobin has a high affinity for oxygen; thus elevated blood sugars prevent the release of oxygen from the red blood cells. The retinal hypoxia that ensues can cause DR to develop or it can exacerbate progression from no retinopathy to subsequent stages of DR. Although evidence now suggests that anemia is also associated with the development of progressive proliferative retinopathy among patients with DM, little attention has been given to anemia as a risk factor for DR in general medical practice. Epidemiologic studies do not exist to support screening for anemia (Bridge & Hirsch); however, anemia is a common health condition of older adults. If anemia is identified in an individual with DM, the health care provider should act quickly to treat the anemia in an effort to prevent DR from developing (Bridge & Hirsch).

As individuals over the age of 65 rarely present without preexisting conditions or diabetes-related comorbidity, the health care provider must consider that management of the older adult is complicated by the population's clinical and functional heterogeneity and that this must be considered when setting diabetes treatment goals (ADA, 2005). Other conditions common to the older adult are coronary artery disease (CAD) and cerebrovascular disease (CVD). Treatment of these conditions often requires that the older adult be placed on aspirin therapy. The Early Treatment Diabetic Retinopathy Study (ETDRS) investigated the effects of aspirin therapy (650 mg/day) on DR. The results of the ETDRS indicated that aspirin use did not affect the progression of retinopathy, it did not increase the risk of developing a vitreous hemorrhage, and it did not increase the duration of a vitreous hemorrhage. There are no ocular contraindications to the use of aspirin therapy when it is required to treat CVD or other medical indications (Fong et al., 2004).

Whenever an older adult is found to have active proliferative retinopathy, that is, actively bleeding vessels, he or she should be discouraged from participating in any activity that increases IOP (Beaser, 2001). The individual should remain active, however, with activities such as walking, swimming, stationary bike riding, and light housekeeping.

Hypertension Management

The Blue Mountains Eye Study examined retinal vessel wall changes resulting from hypertension with a systolic blood pressure ≥ 160 mm Hg or diastolic ≥ 95 mm Hg in a general older population ≥ 49 years of age (Wang et al., 2003). The results of this study support the Beaver Dam Eye Study's findings that retinal hemorrhages and frequent retinal lesion formation in older people without diabetes are significantly related to the formation and presence of arteriolosclerotic plaque as sequela to HTN (Yu, Mitchell, Berry, & Wang, 1998). These and other studies contributed to the establishment of clinical guidelines for the prevention and treatment of HTN. The Seventh Report of the Joint National Committee on Prevention, Detection, Evaluation and Treatment of High Blood Pressure (JNC 7) emphasizes that individuals benefit from BP lowering whether it occurs as a result of lifestyle changes, drug therapies, or from a combination of the two approaches (Joint National Committee, 2004).

The JNC 7 provides classification and detailed categories and criteria for staging BP readings (Table 5.2). The definition of "normal blood pressure" as a systolic BP (SBP) <120 mm Hg and diastolic BP (DBP) <80 mm Hg, is unchanged from the JNC 6 recommendations. A new "prehypertension" category, the most significant change in the classification scheme, has the criteria of a SBP of 120 to 139 mm Hg or DBP 80 to 89 mm Hg. The prehypertension category was designed based on two findings:

1. BP increases steadily with age and most individuals will develop hypertension during their lifetime.
2. Several studies have reported that the mortality rate from vascular diseases, such as cerebrovascular accidents (CVA) and myocardial infarction (MI), increases progressively with a rise in BP levels starting at 115/75 mm Hg (Brookes, 2003).

The guidelines recommend lifestyle changes for prehypertensive individuals as well as for all hypertensive individuals. This should be followed by or in conjunction with pharmacologic agents.

TABLE 5.2 Classification and Management of Blood Pressure in Adults

BP Category	Systolic BP (mm Hg)		Diastolic BP (mm Hg)	Management	Pharmacology*
Normal	<120	and	<80	Lifestyle modification	N/A
Prehypertension	120–139	or	80–89	Lifestyle modification only.	Individuals with DM or renal disease should be placed on ACE or ARB therapy.
Hypertension Stage 1	140–159	or	90–99	BP med(s) and lifestyle modification	Thiazide-type diuretic for most; may consider angiotensin-converting enzyme inhibitor (ACE), angiotensin-receptor blocker (ARB), calcium channel blocker, beta-blocker
Stage 2	>/=160	or	>/=100	Poly BP meds and lifestyle modification	2-drug combination for most (usually thiazide-type diuretic and any of the of the agents above)

*Note: Optimize dosages or add additional drugs until BP goal is met.

Source: Adapted from Joint National Committee, National Heart, Lung, and Blood Institute (2004). The Seventh Report of the Joint National Committee on Prevention, Detection, Evaluation and Treatment of High Blood Pressure (JNC 7). Retrieved May 30, 2005, from http://www.nhlbi.nih.gov/guidelines/hypertension/.

SURGICAL INTERVENTIONS

Panretinal Photocoagulation, Focal Photocoagulation, Vitrectomy

Many therapies have been proposed to prevent or to treat diabetic retinopathy: vitamins, minerals, steroids, bilateral adrenalectomy, hypophysectomy, and radiotherapy. Prior to 1962, pituitary ablation was used in the treatment of proliferative DR (Aiello et al., 1985). In 1962, photocoagulation was introduced; however, it was not until 1976 that the Diabetic Retinopathy Study (DRS) supported the effectiveness of photocoagulation therapy (laser therapy, laser surgery) in the treatment of DR, and photocoagulation became the gold standard for treatment (Aiello et al., 1985). In this study, photocoagulation consisted of panretinal or "scatter" treatment. The National Institutes of Health sponsored the DRS and later the Early Treatment Diabetic Retinopathy Study (ETDRS). These two studies provide the strongest support for photocoagulation surgery when warranted (Aiello et al., 1998). The ETDRS (1979–1989) reaffirmed that scatter treatment significantly reduced severe vision loss when treatment was given early to individuals with proliferative DR (Fong et al., 2004). Furthermore, findings supported deferral of scatter treatment in individuals with mild to moderate nonproliferative DR, until high-risk characteristics (NVD, vitreous hemorrhage with NVE) develop (Fong et al.). The DRS and ETDRS determined that photocoagulation surgery was beneficial in reducing the risk of further visual loss; however, it is not beneficial in reversing any preexisting visual loss (Aiello et al., 1998).

Panretinal Photocoagulation (PRP)

PRP is used to treat proliferative DR. PRP or scatter photocoagulation provides widespread administration of laser by placing burns in a grid pattern across the retina, avoiding the macula and other vital structures (Figure 5.5). This causes extensive peripheral damage while preserving central vision. The laser cauterizes the leaking blood vessels, stops the retina from manufacturing new blood vessels, and causes the proliferating vessels to regress. After undergoing PRP, the older adult should be monitored every 1 to 2 months until the proliferative DR stabilizes.

Focal Photocoagulation

Focal photocoagulation is used to treat mild or moderate nonproliferative DR when microaneurysms or leaking vessels are found within a small area of the retina (Figure 5.6). Focal laser treatment provides a limited number of laser

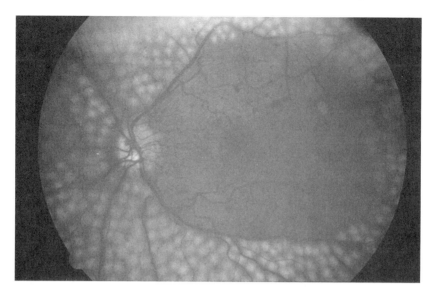

FIGURE 5.5 Panretinal or scatter laser.
Source: National Eye Institute, National Institutes of Health.

beams applied directly to the specific microaneurysm or vessel that cauterizes them, preventing rupture and hemorrhage.

Photocoagulation surgery, both scatter and focal, is now performed in the ophthalmologist's office using an argon laser. Prior to laser surgery, a topical anesthetic is typically applied, and in some individuals a retrobulbar anesthesia may also be given. The pupil is dilated for this procedure as it is with a flourescein scan. The patient is awake during the procedure and sits at a device similar to a slit-lamp. A contact lens is placed on the eye allowing a magnified stereoscopic view of the retina, and an eyelid holder is placed between the lids to prevent blinking. The procedure takes about 30 to 45 minutes to perform. During the procedure, the individual may experience mild discomfort, described as a slight stinging sensation in the eye, and may report seeing brief flashes of light when the laser is being applied. Occasionally individuals will complain that the procedure was painful; however, most are able to tolerate it with little or no adversity. Some individuals may develop a headache or nausea during or after the procedure. The complaint most often reported is that of the need to avoid eye movement by remaining focused on an object during the procedure.

After laser therapy, the older adult will need someone to drive him or her home, as the pupil remains dilated for several hours. The pupil dilation results in photosensitivity, so the older adult should be advised to wear sunglasses

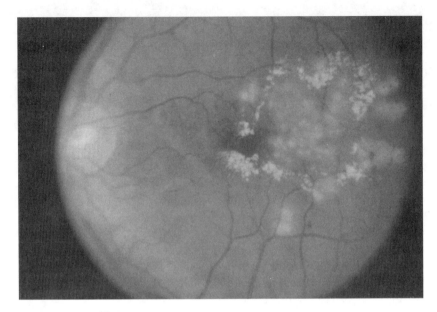

FIGURE 5.6 Focal laser.
Source: National Eye Institute.

to minimize this discomfort. Sometimes the individual complains of blurred vision or eye discomfort for a day or two after laser therapy. This discomfort should be minimal and respond to over-the-counter analgesics.

As with most interventions, there are risks associated with laser therapies. Laser treatment may cause mild loss of central vision, a reduction in night vision, and a decreased ability to focus, and some individuals may lose peripheral vision. In rare instances, a vitreous hemorrhage may develop, causing a traction retinal detachment. There is also the possibility of an accidental laser burn of the fovea resulting in central vision loss. These risks or losses are, however, minimal in comparison to the vision loss that will ensue if DR is left untreated.

Vitrectomy

A vitrectomy involves removal of the vitreous fluid. It is performed to evacuate a vitreous hemorrhage, prevent or repair a retinal detachment, remove scar tissue, and allow treatment of the retina with photocoagulation. The procedure is performed in the hospital setting by a retinal surgeon. The length of the procedure depends on the extent of the repair to be done. The surgeon uses microscopes and special lenses to perform this delicate procedure. Several small incisions are made into the sclera. A fiberoptic light is introduced through one of the incisions to illuminate the area. As fluid is infused through another incision to maintain the shape of the eye, a cutting instrument is introduced through a third to cut and remove the vitreous. Postvitrectomy care varies depending on the extent of repair performed; however, it is typically managed in the outpatient setting and with over-the-counter analgesics.

CONCLUSION

Care of the older adult with DM or HTN presents particular challenges for the health care provider as these conditions can present as insidiously as the retinopathies associated with them. As the numbers of older adults continue to grow, so will the challenge to provide quality, efficient, cost-effective care. Quality and efficient care will be realized by a health care provider who becomes proficient in assessing the older adult for the conditions of DM and HTN and skilled in performing an ophthalmologic exam. The cost-effectiveness of implementing these skills will be realized as a result of early intervention, which can reduce mortality and morbidity.

Over the past decades, there has been much progress made in health care relative to the diagnosis and treatment of DM, HTN, and the retinopathies associated with them. This progress is the result of much evidenced-based research. The result of this research has led to standards of care being established for the treatment of DM and HTN for the purpose of preventing and minimizing co-morbid conditions that may accompany them. It is the challenge of all health care providers to be aware of the latest research findings and standards of care, as these will be the tools utilized to provide quality, efficient, and cost-effective care.

The future holds much promise. Research has shown that it may be possible to reduce the incidence of DM and HTN and associated comorbid conditions. New technologies, medications, and treatments will assist the health care provider in identifying and intervening early in the course of these conditions. It is the responsibility of the health care provider to be knowledgeable about the most current research findings and standards of care for successful management of DM and HTN, to decrease the incidence of vision loss secondary to diabetic and hypertensive retinopathies.

REFERENCES

Albert, D. M., & Dryja, T. P. (1999). The eye. In R. S. Cotran, V. Kumar, T. Collins, & S. L. Robbins (Eds.), *Pathologic basis of disease* (pp. 1368–1370). Philadelphia: Saunders.

Aiello, L. M., Rand, L. I., Sebestyen, J. G., Weiss, J. N., Bradbury, M. J., Wafai, M. Z., & Briones, J. C. (1985). The eyes and diabetes. In E. P. Joslin (Eds.), *Joslin's diabetes mellitus* (pp. 600–634). Philadelphia: Lea & Febiger.

Aiello, L. P., Gardner, T. W., King, G. L., Blankenship, G., Cavallerano, J. D., Ferris, F. L., & Klein, R. (1998). Diabetic retinopathy (Technical Review). *Diabetes Care, 21*, 143–156.

American Diabetes Association (ADA). (2005). American Diabetes Association: Clinical practice recommendations 2004. *Diabetes Care, 28*(Suppl. 1), S4–S36.

Barclay, L. (2002). Telemedicine may improve screening for diabetic retinopathy. *Diabetes Care, 25*(8), 1384–1389. Retrieved April 23, 2004, from http://www.medscape.com/viewwarticle/440571

Beaser, R. S. (2001). Microvascular complications. In R.S. Beaser & the staff of Joslin Diabetes Center (Eds.), *Joslin's diabetes deskbook: A guide for primary care providers* (pp. 373–396). Boston, MA: Joslin Diabetes Center.

Bridge, J., & Hirsch, I. B. (2001). Anemia: A risk factor for diabetic retinopathy? *Practical Diabetology, 20*(4), 32–34.

Brookes, L. (2003, May 14). *The Seventh Report of the Joint National Committee on Prevention, Detection, Evaluation, and the Treatment of High Blood Pressure—NHLBI JNC 7 Press Conference.* Retrieved May 13, 2004, from http://www.medscape.com/viewarticle/455849

Brown, J., Pedula, K. L., & Summers, K. H. (2003). Diabetic retinopathy: Contemporary prevalence in a well-controlled population. *Diabetes Care, 26*(9), 2637–2642.

Ciulla, T. A., Amador, A. G., & Zinman, B. (2003). Diabetic retinopathy and diabetic macular edema. *Diabetes Care, 26*(9), 2653– 2665.

Crawford, J. M., & Cotran, R. S. (1999). The pancreas. In R. S. Cotran, V. Kumar, T. Collins, & S. L. Robbins (Eds.), *Pathologic basis of disease* (pp. 919–920). Philadelphia: Saunders.

Fodera, S. M. (2003). The expanding use of combination therapy in the treatment of hypertension. *Novartis, 17*(2), 1–19.

Fong, D. S., Aiello, L. M., Gardner, T. W., King, G. L., Blankenship, G., Cavallerano, J. D., et al. (2004). American Diabetes Association: Clinical practice recommendations 2004. *Diabetes Care, 27*(Suppl. 1), S84–S87.

Gill, J. M., Cole, D. M., Lebowitz, H. M., & Diamond, J. J. (2004). Accuracy of screening for diabetic retinopathy by family physicians. *Annals of Family Medicine, Inc., 2*(3), 218–220. Retrieved June 25, 2004, from http://www.medscape.com/viewarticle/480051

Joint National Committee, National Heart, Lung, and Blood Institute. (2004). *The Seventh Report of the Joint National Committee on Prevention, Detection, Evaluation and Treatment of High Blood Pressure (JNC 7).* Retrieved May 30, 2005, from http://www.nhlbi.nih.gov/guidelines/hypertension/

Lewis, J. (2003). Prevalence of hypertension among Americans on the rise. *Today in Cardiology.* Retrieved April 23, 2004, from http://www.todayincardiology.com/200310/hypertension.asp?old=never

Lewis, J. (2004). Hypertension often under treated in elderly patients. *Endocrine Today, 2*(7), 25.

Morbidity and Mortality Weekly Report (MMWR). (2004). *Prevalence of diabetes and impaired fasting glucose in adults—United States, 1999–2000* (35th ed., Vol. 52). Retrieved April 23, 2004, from http://www.cdc.gov.mmwr.PDF/wk/mm5235.pdf

National Eye Institute. (2005). Early Treatment Diabetic Retinopathy Study (ETDRS). Message posted to U.S. National Institutes of Health. Retrieved August 20, 2005, from http://www.nei.nih.gov/news/pressreleases/edtrspressrelease.asp

National Eye Institute, U.S. National Institutes of Health. (2005). Retrieved August 1, 2005, from http://www.nei.nih.gov/photo/eyedis/index.asp

Pfeifer, M. A. (1998). Chronic complications of diabetes: An overview. In M. Funnell, C. Hunt, K. Kulkarni, R. Rubin, & P. Yarborough (Eds.), *A core curriculum for diabetes education* (3rd ed., pp. 659–678). Chicago, IL: American Association of Diabetes Educators.

Sowka, J., Gurwood, A. S., & Kabat, A. G. (2001). *Handbook of ocular disease management.* Jobson Publishing. Retrieved April 22, 2004, from http://www.revoptom.com/handbook/SECT41b.HTM

Wang, J., Mitchell, P., Leung, H., Rochtchina, E., Wong, T., & Klein, R. (2003). Hypertensive retinal vessel wall signs in a general older population: The Blue Mountain Eye Study. *Hypertension, 42*(4), 534. Abstract retrieved April 23, 2004, from http://hyper.ahajournals.org/cgi/content/abstract/42/4/534

Wilkinson, C. P. (2003, September 8). *Classification of diabetic retinopathy: A proposed international clinical disease severity grading scale for diabetic retinopathy and diabetic macular edema.* Retrieved November 25, 2003, from http://www.medscape.com/viewprogram/2600_pnt

Yu, T., Mitchell, P., Berry, G., & Wang, J., (1998). Retinopathy in older persons without diabetes and its relations to hypertension. *Epidemiology and Biostatistics, 116*(1), 83–89. Abstract retrieved April 23, 2004, from http://archopht.ama-assn.org/cig/content/abstract/116/1/83

CHAPTER 6

Prevention of Age-Related Vision Loss

Susan Crocker Houde

Research about the prevention of age-related eye disorders provides guidance to the nurse in educating patients and promoting behaviors that may decrease the risk of developing debilitating eye conditions with aging. The nurse may also have a major impact on promoting behaviors that will help delay the progression of vision loss from age-related eye disorders when they do occur. Education is key to enabling individuals to take an active role in promoting eye health.

PREVENTION OF DIABETIC RETINOPATHY

For those with diabetes mellitus, strict control of blood sugars has been shown to decrease both the development and the progression of diabetic retinopathy (Diabetes Control and Complications Trial, 1995). Retinopathy is responsive to prevention of progression through improved blood sugar control and treatment that may delay the onset of loss of vision (Walker, 2004). Education about the relationship between blood sugar control and the development of complications secondary to poor control is an important area for nursing involvement. Nurses may need to become more knowledgeable about the treatment of diabetes so that they may be effective educators of their patients. Patients need to understand the most recent recommendations related to blood sugar control and will need to discuss strategies that will enable them to adhere to their treatment plan. A collaborative relationship between the patient with diabetes and the nurse will maximize the potential for improved blood sugar control.

The progression of diabetic retinopathy is slow and may be silent. Older adults with diabetic retinopathy, therefore, may not realize they are developing the condition unless they have regular screening by an ophthalmologist. Regular eye examinations will detect the condition in its early stages before the patient is aware of its presence. Because diabetic retinopathy has been found in 8% of patients with prediabetes, it is important for all individuals who are diagnosed with diabetes to have an ophthalmological exam on diagnosis (Chamberlain & Janiszewski, 2005). It is also important for all adults to have blood glucose levels checked regularly and to have routine eye examinations to detect diabetes at an early stage. Early detection and treatment is important if permanent vision loss from diabetic retinopathy is to be delayed or prevented. Early treatment has been shown to prevent blindness (Diabetes UK, 2004). The success of interventions to prevent the progression of diabetic retinopathy and the importance of regular screening should be conveyed to patients with diabetes so that fears about vision loss can be decreased and patients have a realistic perception of the outcomes of diabetic retinopathy (National Institute for Clinical Excellence, 2004).

Poor glycemic control has been linked to a decrease in quality of life in research studies (Klein & Klein, 1998). Higher glycemic levels are associated with higher incidences of complications, such as diabetic retinopathy, and may contribute to vision loss. Vision loss has the potential of decreasing functional ability, which in turn may decrease perceptions of quality of life in an older adult. Assessment of functioning in the older adult who is experiencing decreases in vision should assist the nurse in developing interventions that will promote independence and assist the individual in maintaining a high quality of life. The National Eye Institute Visual Functioning Questionnaire 25 (NEI VFQ-25) (Appendix A) is an instrument that may be used to screen older adults for vision loss and issues related to quality of life. Collaborating with older adults to promote and maintain high quality of life in the event of vision loss is an important aspect of the nursing role.

PREVENTION OF CATARACTS

Educating patients about the modifiable risk factors in the development of cataracts may have a positive impact on decreasing the incidence of vision loss worldwide and may promote quality of life in older adults. Possible risk factors in the development of cataracts include advancing age, ultraviolet B radiation, hypertension, smoking, alcohol, deficiency in dietary antioxidants and protein, diabetes, and steroid use (Cumming & Mitchell, 1999; Das, 1999; Gritz, 2001). The Blue Mountain Eye Study found that phenothiazines were associated with nuclear cataracts, aspirin was associated with posterior subcapsular cataracts, and amidarone with cortical cataracts (Cumming & Mitchell, 1998). Results supported that inhaled corticosteroids caused posterior subcapsular cataracts in older adults. The response was found to be dose dependent with a higher incidence in those who used higher doses of inhaled corticosteroids (Cumming & Mitchell, 1999). Patients who are prescribed corticosteroids should be advised of this potential risk of the medication, and attempts should be made to prescribe the lowest possible dose that alleviates symptoms. It is unclear whether different inhaled corticosteroids, with varying potencies, have the same potential for causing cataracts (Cumming & Mitchell, 1999). Future research may provide more insight into the role of inhaled corticosteroids in the development of cataracts.

Sunlight Exposure

Exposure to sunlight may cause damage to the lens and contribute to the development of cataracts. Protection of the eyes from unnecessary radiation from the sun may have an impact on the development of cataracts (Roh & Weiter, 1994). Many adults need education regarding the potential negative effects of sunlight on eye health. Reflective light from the water while boating and snow skiing may also result in cumulative damage. Avoidance of ocular damage from looking at bright lights such as lasers and welding may also be important. Sunglasses that block UV radiation and most blue light are important. The consumer should read labels to be sure they are purchasing protective sunglasses. Sunglasses that fit close to the eyebrow and wrap around the side of the face are more effective in preventing the ultraviolet light rays from entering the eye. Dark sunglasses without UV protection may be hazardous to eye health, as they cause dilation of the pupil, allowing increased transmission of radiation to the eye (Roh & Weiter). Brimmed hats may also be helpful to shield the eye from the harmful effects of the sun.

Cigarette Smoking

Cigarette smoking has been identified as a risk factor for cataracts (Meyer & Sekundo, 2005). The nurse should educate patients about this risk factor. Smoking cessation counseling, suggesting cessation strategies, and referral for support are important nursing role functions with all patients who smoke cigarettes.

Antioxidants

The role of nutrition in eye health is being studied, and antioxidants are emerging as an important component of diet that help to decrease the risk of vision loss from cataracts and age-related macular degeneration (AMD). Lutein and zeaxanthin are not only the major carotenoids in the retina but also the primary carotenoids in the lens. The lifelong effect of sunlight is thought to cause oxidative damage to the lens proteins, leading to the formation of cataracts. Lutein and zeaxanthin absorb ultraviolet light and serve to protect the lens from oxidative damage (Carson & Erdman, 2004). Both the Health Professionals Follow-Up Study and the Nurses' Health Study have demonstrated a decreased risk of lens extraction surgery with lutein and zeaxanthin consumption (Carson & Erdman). Antioxidants in dark, leafy vegetables have been found to protect lens cells from oxidative damage from the sun in the laboratory. This supports the idea that the long-term intake of foods high in lutein and zeaxanthin may have a positive effect on preventing cataracts that are due to oxidative damage (Tufts University, 2005). Higher intake of fruits and vegetables are associated with a lower risk of cataracts in women when followed over a 10-year period (Christen, Liu, Schaumberg, & Buring, 2005).

The role of other antioxidants has been studied related to the prevention of cataracts. The Roche European American Cataract Trial (REACT) demonstrated that those who took 18 mg beta carotene, 750 mg vitamin C, and 600 IU vitamin E for 3 years had a slower progression of lens opacities. Other trials, however, have not demonstrated a beneficial effect of these nutrients on the progression or extraction of lens opacities (Mares, 2004). The results of the Age-Related Eye Disease Study (AREDS) showed that beta carotene, vitamin E, vitamin C, zinc, and copper, when taken in high doses in a supplement, had no impact on the progression of cataracts (Hammond & Johnson, 2002). Generally, clinical trials have supported that b-carotene is not effective in preventing cataracts, and in fact may decrease the absorption of lutein and zeaxanthin (Mares). Vitamin E has also been studied. The administration of 500 IU vitamin E daily over a period of 4 years did not decrease the incidence or progression of nuclear, cortical, or posterior subcapsular cataracts, so the administration of vitamin E is not supported (McNeil et al., 2004). Studies have generally shown that daily multivitamins and the intake of nutrient-rich foods are associated with a lower rate of cataract incidence and cataract extraction. The consumption of high-dose antioxidants in cataract prevention is not supported, however (Mares). Results also seem to support the accumulative protective effects of vitamin supplementation, so that the effects are evident over long periods of time (Mares). A lifetime consuming a diet rich in antioxidants may prevent oxidative damage to the lens. To maximize the intake of lutein and zeaxanthin, a diet rich in fruits and vegetables of various colors should be recommended (Sommerburg, Keunen, Bird, & Van Kuijk, 1998). Table 6.1 provides an overview of foods that are high in lutein and zeaxanthin to guide the nurse and patient. Beginning a nutrient-rich diet later in life, when oxidative damage has already occurred, may not be effective in retarding

TABLE 6.1 Foods High in Lutein and Zeaxanthin

Spinach
Kale
Turnip greens
Mustard greens
Dandelion greens
Summer squash (all varieties)
Peas
Noodles (egg or spinach)
Winter squash (all varieties)
Broccoli
Beet greens
Pumpkin
Sweet peppers
Corn—yellow
Brussel sprouts
Lettuce
Cornmeal
Eggs[a]
Onions
Beans—yellow and green snap
Orange juice

Source: Adapted from USDA Nutrient Data Laboratory. *USDA National Nutrient Database for Standard Reference*, Release 17. Retrieved May 13, 2006, from www.nal.usda.gov/fnic/foodcomp/Data/SR17/wtrank/sr17w338.pdf
[a]Egg yolks are also a good source of lutein and zeaxanthin and can easily be prepared and consumed by older adults. Research has demonstrated that consuming one egg per day increases levels of lutein and zeaxanthin in the blood (Goodrow, Wilson, Houde, Vishwanathan, Scollin, Handelman, & Nicolosi, 2006).

progression of cataracts (Hammond & Johnson). There is still some confusion as to the effect of specific nutrients on the development and progression of cataracts. Further research will clarify the role of nutrients on this common eye condition, which is the leading cause of blindness worldwide.

PREVENTION OF AGE-RELATED MACULAR DEGENERATION

Several of the modifiable risk factors for cataracts are also risk factors for the development of AMD. As with cataracts, AMD is thought to be due to long-term oxidative damage to the retina. Modifiable risk factors for AMD include smoking, hypertension, low dietary intake of carotenoids, low serum zinc levels, lifetime sunlight exposure, elevated cholesterol level, hyperopia, excessive alcohol consumption, cardiovascular disease, lack of postmenopausal estrogen use, and physical inactivity (Pratt, 1999). Nonmodifiable risk factors include: increasing age, family history of AMD, female gender, light-colored irises, and increased parity (Pratt). Age has been identified as a strong nonmodifiable risk factor. In a combined analysis of three major eye studies in three continents, AMD was found in 0.2% of those ages 55 to 64 and in 13% of those adults over the age of 85 (Smith et al., 2001).

Antioxidants

The use of antioxidants in the prevention of vision loss from AMD continues to be studied. Important results from the AREDS trial demonstrated that individuals with intermediate AMD or advanced AMD in one eye, benefited from the intake of antioxidant supplements with high doses of zinc, copper, vitamins C and E, and beta carotene. The benefit of combined antioxidant and zinc intake was a 5% to 30% reduction in the progression to advanced AMD (Jampol, 2001). A decrease in progression was not found in those with early AMD because the rate of progression in the control group was very small. No adverse effects of the supplementation were noted. The doses used in the trial were much larger than those found in over-the-counter vitamin supplements (500 mg vitamin C, 400 IU vitamin E, 80 mg zinc, 15 mg beta-carotene, and 2 mg of cupric oxide). One should use caution in recommending beta-carotene in smokers or recent ex-smokers because beta-carotene has been associated with a greater risk of lung cancer in this population (The Alpha-Tocopherol, Beta Carotene Cancer Prevention Study Group, 1994). There is also little evidence that vitamin E alone has a protective effect against AMD (Hall & Gale, 2002).

Lutein and Zeaxanthin

Many studies have been conducted that examine the relationship between consuming fruits, vegetables, and vitamins and the development and progression of AMD. There has been focus on the role of carotenoids and AMD. Interest has been focused recently on lutein and zeaxanthin, the two dominant carotenoids in the macular pigment. Many people have a low concentration of macular pigment, and this may contribute to negative visual effects (Stringham & Hammond, 2005). Research has demonstrated a relationship between lutein and zeaxanthin intake in the diet, serum levels of lutein and zeaxanthin, and macular pigment density (Curran-Celentano, Hammond, Ciulla, Cooper, Pratt, & Danis, 2001). Improvement in macular pigment density has been associated with improvement in vision for those with and without AMD, and may have a protective effect against the development and progression of AMD.

Lutein and zeaxanthin are found in a number of bright green, orange, and yellow vegetables (Table 6.1), as well as in vitamin supplements. The average American consumes approximately 1 to 2 mg of lutein daily. In the Lutein Antioxidant Supplementation Trial (LAST), ingesting 10 mg of a lutein supplement or a supplement mix of antioxidants resulted in a 50% increase in ocular pigment density compared to placebo as well as an improvement in visual acuity, glare recovery, and contrast sensitivity (Richer et al., 2004).

Results have generally been supportive of the protective nature of fruits and vegetables. A recent study, however, did not find an association between the consumption of vegetables rich in lutein and zeaxanthin or vitamin supplements, and AMD. The results of the study did support that the consumption of fruits were protective, and those who ate three or more servings of fruit per day had a 36% reduced risk of developing AMD compared to those who ate fewer than 1.5 servings per day (Cho, Seddon, Rosner, Willett, & Hankinson, 2004). It was hypothesized that nutrients in fruits, other than lutein and zeaxanthin, may have a positive effect on preventing AMD.

Education for patients and the general public about the importance of eating a well-balanced diet, with plenty of green leafy, orange, and yellow vegetables, as well as several servings of fruit daily may have a positive influence on preventing vision loss in old age. The nurse's role in advocacy for lifelong healthy eating to promote health is important when communicating with patients of all ages.

Cigarette Smoking

Cigarette smoking has been identified as the principle preventable risk factor associated with AMD. Researchers examined results of several large studies focusing on AMD, including the Beaver Dam Eye Study in the United States, the Blue Mountain Eye Study in Australia, and the Rotterdam Eye Study in Europe, and each study demonstrated a significant relationship between smoking and AMD (Guttman, 2003; Smith, Seligsohn, Khan, & Spaeth, 2001). When combining data from the three studies, those who were current smokers had a 300-fold increased risk of developing AMD. The risk for AMD decreased with the cessation of smoking, but remained substantially higher than for those who had never smoked (Guttman; Smith et al.). In a study of 4,000 adults ages 75 and older in the United Kingdom, those who were smokers were twice as likely to be diagnosed with AMD as nonsmokers (Evans, Fletcher, & Wormald, 2005). Twenty years after having stopped smoking, the risk of developing AMD decreased to the level of those who had never smoked and some reduction in risk was seen after 10 years (Evans, Fletcher, & Wormald).

Educating smokers of all ages related to the increased incidence of AMD in those who smoke is important. The risk of smoking in the development of lung cancer and cardiovascular disease is well known by the general public. The increased risk in smokers of developing AMD, the leading cause of blindness in well-developed countries, is less well known. Nurses should play a leading role in educating patients and the general public about this important risk factor. Knowledge about this important risk factor, and the fear of losing vision as one ages, may be an important deterrent to those who smoke and those at risk for becoming a smoker in the future.

Sunlight Exposure

It is also important to educate patients and the general public about the role of lifetime exposure to sunlight in the development of AMD. In a 10-year study, it was found that those who were exposed to summer sunlight for extended periods of time in their teens and 30s were more likely to develop AMD at an early age. In those that reported the highest amount of sun exposure, a protective effect of wearing a hat and sunglasses was found (Tomany, Cruickshanks, Klein, Klein, & Knudtson, 2004).

Fats, Cholesterol, and Fish Intake

Another area that has been explored is the role of fat, cholesterol, and fish intake on the development of AMD. Higher intakes of cholesterol, linoleic acid, vegetable, monosaturated, and polyunsaturated fat have been associated with an increased risk of developing advanced AMD (Seddon et al., 2001; Smith, Mitchell, & Leeder, 2000). Animal fats have been associated with an increase in progression of AMD, but the intake of vegetable fats has shown a stronger relationship with progression of the disorder (Seddon, Cote, & Rosner, 2003). Total and saturated fat intake have been associated with a borderline increase in developing early AMD (Smith, Mitchell, & Leeder). Fish intake has been shown to have a protective effect against AMD in some studies. One study found that those who had a low intake of linoleic acid and a diet that was high in fish and omega-3 fatty acids were less likely to develop advanced AMD (Seddon et al.). Others found a protective effect of eating fresh or frozen fish at low levels of intake, but no increase in protection with greater levels of fish consumption (Smith, Mitchell, & Leeder). Nuts have also been found to have a protective effect on the progression of AMD (Seddon, Cote, & Rosner).

Education about healthy eating is important, not only for the prevention of cardiovascular disease but also for the prevention of vision loss related to AMD. Diets that are low in fats may contribute to eye health. Processed baked goods have been associated with the progression of AMD (Seddon, Cote, & Rosner, 2003). Education related to decreasing the fat in baked goods and preparing baked goods using low-fat methodologies may be important for cardiovascular and eye health. Low-fat diets that have been promoted for cardiovascular health for years may also be helpful in promoting eye health. Further research is needed to understand the relationship between fats in the diet and AMD, but data support that healthy eating practices, including low-fat diets that are high in antioxidants, may be important to maintain good vision.

Statins and Aspirin Therapy

There has been conflicting evidence on the effectiveness of statin and aspirin therapy in preventing the progression of AMD. There are studies that have supported their protective role against AMD (McGwin, Owsley, Curcio, & Crain, 2003; Wilson, Schwartz, Bhatt, McCulloch, & Duncan, 2004), and others that have not supported a positive role for the medications (Klein, Klein, Tomany, Danforth, & Cruickshanks, 2003; Van Leeuwen, Vingerling, Hofman, De Jong, & Stricker, 2003). In a randomized trial study of physicians, researchers found no statistically significant protective effect of 5 years of low-dose aspirin therapy on the development of AMD (Christen et al., 2001). It has been postulated that the reason for the discrepancy in results is related to limitations in study designs, and that further study is necessary before resolving the issue of whether statins or aspirin have a positive effect on the development or progression of AMD (Klein & Klein, 2004). Nurses should continue to follow current research in this area, as it is too early to draw any conclusions from the existing data.

PREVENTION OF GLAUCOMA

The nurse can have a positive impact on motivating the patient with modifiable risk factors to make positive changes on behaviors that can reduce risk of developing glaucoma with advancing age. Modifiable risk factors include cigarette smoking and increased intraocular pressure (Aref & Schmitt, 2005). Cigarette smoking as a risk factor has been controversial in the past, but the results of a recent meta-analysis supports cigarette smoking as being an important risk factor in the development of primary open-angle glaucoma (Bonovas, Filioussi, Tsantes, & Peponis, 2004). Educating patients about the association between cigarette smoking and the development of glaucoma and the provision of smoking cessation counseling and referral may provide the impetus to patients for positive change.

The best way to prevent vision loss from glaucoma is to encourage regular screening for glaucoma, so that treatment can be started before vision loss occurs. Educating the patient about the importance of regular screening for glaucoma, even if asymptomatic, is important. It is recommended that patients ages 40 to 60 have regular eye exams every 2 years; and those over 60 years old, annually (Smith et al., 2004). It is important to identify those individuals with elevations in intraocular pressure, as elevations in intraocular pressure can be treated and monitored, increasing the chance of avoiding vision loss in old age. Those at risk for developing glaucoma, including diabetics, those with a family history of glaucoma in a first-degree relative, African Americans, and those who have used steroids long term should be screened for glaucoma annually beginning at a younger age.

The leading cause of blindness in African Americans is glaucoma. Topical ocular hypotensive therapy has been shown to be effective in preventing and delaying the onset of glaucoma in a sample of African Americans with ocular hypertension (Higginbotham et al., 2004). This preventative treatment may be an option if the patient has a high probability of developing glaucoma because of the presence of ocular hypertension and additional risk factors. Decreasing intraocular pressure has been shown to decrease the progression of visual field loss (The AGIS Investigators, 2000). Nurses should educate patients about the need for the identification of risk factors and the early detection of glaucoma so that treatment can be initiated and vision loss can be prevented.

CONCLUSION

The nurse has a challenging role in educating patients and the general public about risk factors and strategies to prevent vision loss from age-related eye disorders. It is important that the nurse keep informed about current scientific evidence that is evolving in this exciting area of prevention of eye disorders in older adults. Sharing results of research related to risk factors and preventative strategies is important in order for patients to make informed decisions about changing behaviors that may benefit eye health and vision in later years. Assessing and monitoring progression of visual loss, while attempting to prevent further vision loss through preventative interventions, is an important aspect of the nursing role. Referral to eye specialists, identifying resources, and educating both patients and families about preventative strategies may be important in assisting patients to cope with their diagnosis and to take an active role in preventing the progression of their eye disorder. Maintaining eye health through preventative strategies will have a positive impact on the quality of life for older adults.

REFERENCES

Aref, A., & Schmitt, B. (2005). Open-angle glaucoma: Tips for earlier detection and treatment selection. *Journal of Family Practice, 54*(2), 117–125.

Bonovas, S., Filioussi, K., Tsantes, A., & Peponis, V. (2004). Epidemiological association between cigarette smoking and primary open-angle glaucoma: A meta-analysis. *Public Health, 118*(4), 256–261.

Carson, L., & Erdman, J. (2004). Carotenoids and eye health. *Nutrition and the M.D. 30*(3), 1–4.

Chamberlain, J., & Janiszewski, R. (2005). Diabetic retinopathy occurs in pre-diabetes. *NIH News*. Retrieved August 8, 2005, from http://www.nih.gov/news/pr/june2005/niddk-12.htm

Cho, E., Seddon, J., Rosner, B., Willett, W., & Hankinson, S. (2004). Prospective study of intake of fruits, vegetables, vitamins, and carotenoids and risk of age-related maculopathy. *Archives of Ophthalmology, 122*(6), 883–892.

Christen, W. G., Liu, S., Schaumberg, D. A., & Buring, J. E. (2005). Fruit and vegetable intake and the risk of cataract in women. *American Journal of Clinical Nutrition, 81*(6), 1417–1422.

Christen, W., Glynn, R., Ajani, U., Schaumberg, D., Chew, E., Buring, J., et al. (2001). Age-related maculopathy in a randomized trial of low-dose aspirin among US physicians. *Archives of Ophthalmology, 119*(8), 1143–1149.

Cumming, R. G., & Mitchell, P. (1998). Medications and cataract: The Blue Mountain Eye Study. *Ophthalmology, 105*(9), 1751–1758.

Cumming, R. G., & Mitchell, P. (1999). Inhaled corticosteroids and cataract: Prevalence, prevention and management. *Drug Safety, 20*(1), 77–84.

Curran-Celentano, J., Hammond, B., Ciulla, T., Cooper, D., Pratt, L., & Danis, R. (2001). Relationship between dietary intake, serum concentrations, and retinal concentrations of lutein and zeaxanthin in adults in a midwest population. *American Journal of Clinical Nutrition, 74*(6), 796–802.

Das, A. (1999). Prevention of vision loss in older adults. *Clinics in Geriatric Medicine, 15*(1), 131–135.

Diabetes Control and Complications Trial. (1995). The effect of intensive diabetes treatment on the progression of diabetic retinopathy in insulin dependent diabetes mellitus. *Archives of Ophthalmology, 113*(1), 36–51.

Diabetes UK. (2004). *Diabetes in the UK 2004*. London: Diabetes UK.

Evans, J., Fletcher, A., & Wormald, R. (2005). 28,000 cases of age related macular degeneration causing visual loss in people aged 75 years and above in the United Kingdom may be attributable to smoking. *British Journal of Ophthalmology, 89*, 550–553.

Goodrow, E., Wilson, T., Houde, S., Vishwanathan, R., Scollin, P., Handelman, G., & Nicolosi, R. (2006). Consumption of one egg per day increases serum lutein and zeaxanthin in older adults without altering serum lipid and lipoprotein cholesterol concentrations. *Journal of Nutrition* (in press).

Gritz, D. (2001). Can cataracts be prevented? *Bulletin of the World Health Organization,* *79*(3), 260–261.

Guttman, C. (2003). Smoke alarm: New analyses strengthen link between smoking and AMD. *Ophthalmology Times, 28*(8), 1.

Hall, N., & Gale, C. (2002). Prevention of age related macular degeneration: Current evidence suggests that vitamin E alone is unlikely to have a large protective effect. *British Medical Journal, 325*(7354), 1–2.

Hammond, B. R., & Johnson, M. A. (2002). The Age-related Eye Disease Study (AREDS). *Nutrition Reviews, 60*(9), 283–288.

Higginbotham, E., Gordon, M., Beiser, J., Drake, M., Bennett, G., Wilson, M., et al. (2004). The Ocular Hypertension Treatment Study: Topical medication delays or prevents primary open-angle glaucoma in African American individuals. *Archives of Ophthalmology, 122*(6), 813–820.

Jampol, L. M. (2001). Antioxidants, zinc, and age-related macular degeneration. *Archives of Ophthalmology, 119*(10), 1533–1534.

Klein, R., & Klein, B. (1998). Relation of glycemic control to diabetic complications and health outcomes. *Diabetic Care, 21*(Suppl. 3), C39–C43.

Klein, R., & Klein, B. (2004). Do statins prevent age-related macular degeneration? *American Journal of Ophthalmology, 137*(4), 747–749.

Klein, R., Klein, B., Tomany, S., Danforth, L., & Cruickshanks, K. (2003). Relation of statin use to the 5-year incidence and progression of age-related maculopathy. *Archives of Ophthalmology, 121*(8), 1151–1155.

Mares, J. (2004). High-dose antioxidant supplementation and cataract risk. *Nutrition Reviews, 62*(1), 28–32.

McGwin, G., Jr., Owsley, C., Curcio, C., & Crain, R. (2003). The association between statin use and age related maculopathy. *British Journal of Ophthalmology, 87,* 1121–1125.

McNeil, J., Robman, L., Tikellis, G., Sinclair, M., McCarty, C., & Taylor, H. (2004). Vitamin E supplementation and cataract—A randomized trial. *Ophthalmology, 111*(1), 75–84.

Meyer, C. H., & Sekundo, W. (2005). Nutritional supplementation to prevent cataract formation. *Developments in Ophthalmology, 38,* 103–119.

National Institute for Clinical Excellence. (2004). *Type 1 diabetes: Diagnosis and management of type 1 diabetes in children, young people, and adults.* Clinical Guideline 15. London: NICE.

Pratt, S. (1999). Dietary prevention of age-related macular degeneration. *Journal of the American Optometric Association, 70*(1), 39–47.

Richer, S., Stiles, W., Statkute, L., Pulido, J., Frankowski, J., Rudy, D., et al. (2004). Double-masked, placebo-controlled, randomized trial of lutein and antioxidant supplementation in the intervention of atrophic age-related macular degeneration: The Veterans LAST study. *Optometry: Journal of American Optometric Association, 75*(4), 216–230.

Roh, S., & Weiter, J. J. (1994). Light damage to the eye. *Journal of the Florida Medical Association, 81*(4), 248–251.

Seddon, J., Cote, J., & Rosner, B. (2003). Progression of age-related macular degeneration: Association with dietary fat, transunsaturated fat, and fish intake. *Archives of Ophthalmology, 121*(12), 1728–1737.

Seddon, J., Rosner, B., Sperduto, R., Yannuzzi, L., Haller, J., Blair, N., & Willett, W. (2001). Dietary fat and risk for advanced age-related macular degeneration. *Archives of Ophthalmology, 119*(8), 1191–1199.

Smith, W., Assink, J., Klein, R., Mitchell, P., Klaver, C., Klein, B., et al. (2001). Risk factors for age-related macular degeneration: Pooled findings from three continents. *Ophthalmology, 108*, 697–704.

Smith, O., Seligsohn, A., Khan, S., & Spaeth, G. (2004). *Primary open-angle glaucoma.* American College of Physicians PIER Guideline.

Smith, W., Mitchell, P., & Leeder, S. (2000). Dietary fat and fish intake and age-related maculopathy. *Archives of Ophthalmology, 118*, 401–404.

Sommerburg, O., Keunen, J., Bird, A., & Van Kuijk, F. (1998). Fruits and vegetables are sources for lutein and zeaxanthin: The macular pigment in human eyes. *British Journal of Ophthalmology, 82*(8), 907–910.

Stringham J., & Hammond, B. (2005). Dietary lutein and zeaxanthin: Possible effects on visual function. *Nutrition Reviews, 63*(2), 59–64.

The AGIS Investigators. (2000). The Advanced Glaucoma Intervention Study (AGIS): The relationship between control of intraocular pressure and visual field deterioration. *American Journal of Ophthalmology, 130*(4), 429–440.

The Alpha-Tocopherol, Beta Carotene Cancer Prevention Study Group. (1994). The effects of vitamin E and beta carotene on the incidence of lung cancer and other cancers in smokers. *New England Journal of Medicine, 330*, 1029–1035.

Tomany, S., Cruickshanks, K., Klein, R., Klein, B., & Knudtson, M. (2004). Sunlight and the 10-year incidence of age-related maculopathy: The Beaver Dam Eye Study. *Archives of Ophthalmology, 122*(5), 750–757.

Tufts University. (2005). Antioxidants from dark, leafy greens protects against cataracts. *Tufts University Health and Nutrition Letter, 23*(1), 2.

USDA Nutrient Data Laboratory. *USDA National Nutrient Database for Standard Reference*, Release 17. Retrieved May 13, 2006, from www.nal.usda.gov/fnic/foodcomp/Data/SR17/wtrank/sr17w338.pdf

Van Leeuwen, R., Vingerling, J., Hofman, A., De Jong, P., & Stricker, B. (2003). Cholesterol lowering drugs and the risk of age related maculopathy: Prospective cohort study with cumulative exposure measurement. *British Medical Journal, 326*(7383), 255–256.

Walker, R. (2004). Diabetic retinopathy: Protecting the vision of people with diabetes. *British Journal of Community Nursing, 9*(12), 545–547.

Wilson, H., Schwartz, D., Bhatt, H., McCulloch, C., & Duncan, J. (2004). Statin and aspirin therapy are associated with decreased rates of choroidal neovascularization among patients with age-related macular degeneration. *American Journal of Ophthalmology, 137*(4), 615–624.

APPENDIX A: NATIONAL EYE INSTITUTE, VISUAL FUNCTIONING QUESTIONNAIRE-25 (VFQ-25)

Instructions:

I'm going to read you some statements about problems that involve your vision or feelings that you have about your vision condition. After each question I will read you a list of possible answers. Please choose the response that best describes your situation.

Please answer all the questions as if you were wearing your glasses or contact lenses (if any).

PART 1 - GENERAL HEALTH AND VISION

1. *In general*, would you say your overall *health* is:

(Circle One)

READ CATEGORIES:
Excellent 1
Very Good 2
Good 3
Fair 4
Poor 5

2. At the present time, would you say your eyesight using both eyes (with glasses or contact lenses, if you wear them) is *excellent, good, fair, poor*, or *very poor* or are you *completely blind*?

(Circle One)

READ CATEGORIES:
Excellent 1
Good 2
Fair 3
Poor 4
Very Poor 5
Completely Blind 6

3. How much of the time do you *worry* about your eyesight?

(Circle One)

READ CATEGORIES:
None of the time 1
A little of the time 2
Some of the time 3
Most of the time 4
All of the time? 5

4. How much *pain or discomfort* have you had *in and around your eyes* (for example, burning, itching, or aching)? Would you say it is:

(*Circle One*)

READ CATEGORIES:

None 1
Mild 2
Moderate 3
Severe 4
Very severe? 5

PART 2 - DIFFICULTY WITH ACTIVITIES

The next questions are about how much difficulty, if any, you have doing certain activities wearing your glasses or contact lenses if you use them for that activity.

5. How much difficulty do you have *reading ordinary print in newspapers*? Would you say you have:

(READ CATEGORIES AS NEEDED)

(*Circle One*)

No difficulty at all 1
A little difficulty 2
Moderate difficulty 3
Extreme difficulty 4
Stopped doing this because of your eyesight 5
Stopped doing this for other reasons or not interested in doing this 6

6. How much difficulty do you have doing work or hobbies that require you to *see well up close*, such as cooking, sewing, fixing things around the house, or using hand tools? Would you say:

(READ CATEGORIES AS NEEDED)

(*Circle One*)

No difficulty at all 1
A little difficulty 2
Moderate difficulty 3
Extreme difficulty 4
Stopped doing this because of your eyesight 5
Stopped doing this for other reasons or not interested in doing this 6

7. Because of your eyesight, how much difficulty do you have *finding something on a crowded shelf?*

(READ CATEGORIES AS NEEDED)

(Circle One)

No difficulty at all 1
A little difficulty 2
Moderate difficulty 3
Extreme difficulty 4
Stopped doing this because of your eyesight 5
Stopped doing this for other reasons or not interested in doing this 6

8. How much difficulty do you have *reading street signs or the names of stores?*

(READ CATEGORIES AS NEEDED)

(Circle One)

No difficulty at all 1
A little difficulty 2
Moderate difficulty 3
Extreme difficulty 4
Stopped doing this because of your eyesight 5
Stopped doing this for other reasons or not interested in doing this 6

9. Because of your eyesight, how much difficulty do you have *going down steps, stairs, or curbs in dim light or at night?*

(READ CATEGORIES AS NEEDED)

(Circle One)

No difficulty at all 1
A little difficulty 2
Moderate difficulty 3
Extreme difficulty 4
Stopped doing this because of your eyesight 5
Stopped doing this for other reasons or not interested in doing this 6

10. Because of your eyesight, how much difficulty do you have *noticing objects off to the side while you are walking along?*

(READ CATEGORIES AS NEEDED)

(Circle One)

No difficulty at all 1
A little difficulty 2
Moderate difficulty 3

Extreme difficulty 4
Stopped doing this because of your eyesight 5
Stopped doing this for other reasons or not interested in doing this 6

11. Because of your eyesight, how much difficulty do you have *seeing how people react to things* you say?

(READ CATEGORIES AS NEEDED)

(Circle One)

No difficulty at all 1
A little difficulty 2
Moderate difficulty 3
Extreme difficulty 4
Stopped doing this because of your eyesight 5
Stopped doing this for other reasons or not interested in
    doing this 6

12. Because of your eyesight, how much difficulty do you have *picking out and matching your own clothes*?

(READ CATEGORIES AS NEEDED)

(Circle One)

No difficulty at all 1
A little difficulty 2
Moderate difficulty 3
Extreme difficulty 4
Stopped doing this because of your eyesight 5
Stopped doing this for other reasons or not interested in
    doing this 6

13. Because of your eyesight, how much difficulty do you have *visiting with people in their homes, at parties, or in restaurants*?

(READ CATEGORIES AS NEEDED)

(Circle One)

No difficulty at all 1
A little difficulty 2
Moderate difficulty 3
Extreme difficulty 4
Stopped doing this because of your eyesight 5
Stopped doing this for other reasons or not interested in
    doing this 6

14. Because of your eyesight, how much difficulty do you have *going out to see movies, plays, or sports events*?

(READ CATEGORIES AS NEEDED)
(Circle One)

No difficulty at all 1
A little difficulty 2
Moderate difficulty 3
Extreme difficulty 4
Stopped doing this because of your eyesight 5
Stopped doing this for other reasons or not interested in
    doing this 6

15. Now, I'd like to ask about *driving a car*. Are you *currently driving*, at least once in a while?

(Circle One)
Yes 1   *Skip To Q 15c*
No 2

15a. IF NO, ASK: Have you *never* driven a car or have you *given up driving*

(Circle One)
Never drove 1   *Skip To Part 3, Q 17*
Gave up 2

15b. IF GAVE UP DRIVING: Was that *mainly because of your eyesight, mainly for some other reason*, or because of *both your eyesight and other reasons*?

(Circle One)
Mainly eyesight 1   *Skip To Part 3, Q 17*
Mainly other reasons 2   *Skip To Part 3, Q 17*
Both eyesight and other reasons . . 3   *Skip To Part 3, Q 17*

15c. IF CURRENTLY DRIVING: How much difficulty do you have *driving during the daytime in familiar places*? Would you say you have:

(Circle One)
No difficulty at all 1
A little difficulty 2
Moderate difficulty 3
Extreme difficulty 4

16.   How much difficulty do you have *driving at night*? Would you say you have:

(READ CATEGORIES AS NEEDED)
(Circle One)

No difficulty at all 1
A little difficulty 2
Moderate difficulty 3
Extreme difficulty 4
Have you stopped doing this because
    of your eyesight 5
Have you stopped doing this for other
    reasons or are you not interested in
    doing this 6

16a.   How much difficulty do you have *driving in difficult conditions, such as in bad weather, during rush hour, on the freeway, or in city traffic*? Would you say you have:

(READ CATEGORIES AS NEEDED)
(Circle One)

No difficulty at all 1
A little difficulty 2
Moderate difficulty 3
Extreme difficulty 4
Have you stopped doing this because
    of your eyesight 5
Have you stopped doing this for other
    reasons or are you not interested in
    doing this 6

PART 3: RESPONSES TO VISION PROBLEMS

The next questions are about how things you do may be affected by your vision. For each one, I'd like you to tell me if this is true for you *all*, *most*, *some*, *a little*, or *none* of the time.

	(Circle One On Each Line)				
READ CATEGORIES:	All of the time	Most of the time	Some of the time	A little of the time	None of the time
17. *Do you accomplish less* than you would like because of your vision?	1	2	3	4	5

18. *Are you limited* in how long you
can work or do other activities
because of your vision?   1   2   3   4   5

19. How much does pain or
discomfort *in or around your eyes*,
for example, burning, itching, or
aching, keep you from doing what
you'd like to be doing? Would you
say: 1   2   3   4   5

For each of the following statements, please tell me if it is *definitely true*, *mostly true*, *mostly false*, or *definitely false* for you or you are *not sure*.

	(Circle One On Each Line)				
	Definitely True	Mostly True	Not Sure	Mostly False	Definitely False
20. I *stay home most of the time* because of my eyesight.	1	2	3	4	5
21. I feel *frustrated* a lot of the time because of my eyesight.	1	2	3	4	5
22. I have *much less control* over what I do, because of my eyesight.	1	2	3	4	5
23. Because of my eyesight, I have to *rely too much on what other people tell me*.	1	2	3	4	5
24. I *need a lot of help* from others because of my eyesight.	1	2	3	4	5
25. I worry about *doing things that will embarrass myself or others*, because of my eyesight.	1	2	3	4	5

Source: RAND. (2000). National Eye Institute Visual Functioning Questionnaire 25 (VFQ-25). Developed at RAND under the sponsorship of the National Eye Institute. Permission granted by RAND Corporation, Santa Monica, Calif., www.rand.org/publications/health, for use of instrument.

CHAPTER 7

Psychological and Social Impact of Age-Related Vision Loss

Karen Devereaux Melillo

Vision loss of any type is a dramatic event in the life of older adults. Whether acute or gradual in onset, partial (low vision) or full (blindness), any vision change can threaten the basic need for functional independence that elders so actively seek to maintain. Visual impairment is 1 of the 10 most frequent causes of disability in the United States (U.S. Department of Health and Human Services [USDHHS], 2001). For individuals age 70 and older, 18.1% report vision impairments (Campbell, Crews, Moriarty, Zack, & Blackman, 1999). As age increases, the percentage of adults with vision loss increases (Pleis & Coles, 2003).

In addition to the increased incidence of vision loss with advancing age, eye conditions and visual impairment also vary by race/ethnicity, gender, and socioeconomic status. Data from the 1999 National Health Interview Survey reported that for the U.S. adult population in general, vision impairment with corrective lenses is reported in 5% of Asian adults, 8% of Black adults, 9% White adults, and 11% American Indian or Alaska Native adults. Also, non-Hispanic White and non-Hispanic Black adults are more likely to have vision difficulty than are Hispanic adults (Pleis & Coles, 2003). In a study of vision impairment among elderly African Americans ($n = 998$), 36.5% described their vision as either fair (21.4%) or poor (15.1%) (Bazargan, Baker, & Bazargan, 2001).

Women are slightly more likely to have experienced vision loss than men, and 14% of adults who had family incomes below the poverty threshold experienced vision problems compared with 8% of adults whose family income was at least two times greater than the poverty threshold (Pleis & Coles, 2003).

These statistics speak to the need to promote policies that assure access to and availability of preventive vision care and vision rehabilitation services for older adults in general and vulnerable groups in particular.

Vision loss can impact an older adult's perceived quality of life by affecting basic and instrumental activities of daily living, psychological well-being, and social interactions. The psychological and social coping and adaptation of older adults to their visual impairment, as well as the major contributions that the environment and public policy play in this process, is the focus of this chapter.

Healthy People 2010 has identified among its goals the need to "improve the visual . . . health of the Nation through prevention, early detection, treatment, and rehabilitation" (USDHHS, 2001, Section 28). When vision loss does occur, however, an older adult must adapt to the impairment, activity limitation, or participation restriction that can ensue as a result, as well as cope with health and health-related outcomes. For older adults, *Healthy People 2010* suggests that increasing access to and use of vision rehabilitation is one of the objectives designed to achieve this goal and, as a result, to foster psychological and social adjustment to vision loss.

PSYCHOLOGICAL IMPACT

A number of researchers have noted that adaptation to age-related vision loss is affected by knowledge of and access to rehabilitation services, functionality, and support received from one's social network, as well as by the use of coping strategies (Brennan, 2002; Brennan et al., 2001). The World Health Organization (WHO, 2001) has developed the *International Classification of Functioning, Disability and Health* that can serve as a model for understanding the psychological and social impact of vision loss. As presented in Table 7.1, Part 1 reflects the actual functioning and disability experienced due to vision loss, whereas Part 2 addresses the contextual factors, both environmental and personal, that can positively or negatively influence adaptation and coping. In particular, the WHO notes, "a person's functioning and disability is conceived as a dynamic interaction between health conditions [i.e., vision loss] and contextual factors . . . both personal and environmental" (p. 8). WHO further defines environmental factors as those physical, social, and attitudinal components that make up where people live and how they conduct their lives. Personal factors include "gender, race, age, other health conditions, fitness, lifestyle, habits, upbringing, coping styles, social background, education, profession, past and current experience, overall behavior pattern and character style, individual psychological assets and other characteristics" (p. 17). The nurse who holistically assesses individuals with vision loss

TABLE 7.1 Overview of the International Classification of Functioning, Disability, and Health

	Part 1: Functioning and Disability		Part 2: Contextual Factors	
Components	Body functions and structures	Activities and participation	Environmental factors	Personal factors
Domains	Body functions Body structures	Life areas (tasks, actions)	External influences on functioning and disability	Internal influences on functioning and disability
Constructs	Change in body functions (physiological) Change in body structures (anatomical)	Capacity Executing tasks in a standard environment Performance Executing tasks in the current environment	Facilitating or hindering impact of features of the physical, social, and attitudinal world	Impact of attributes of the person
Positive aspect	Functional and structural integrity	Activities participation	Facilitators	Not applicable
	Functioning			
Negative aspect	Impairment	Activity limitation Participation restriction	Barriers/hindrances	Not applicable
	Disability			

Source: From World Health Organization. (2001). International classification of functioning, disability, and health. Retrieved July 7, 2004, from http://WHO.int/classification/icf/imtros/ICF-Eng-Intro.pdf. Reprinted with permission from WHO.

111

recognizes that these variables can impact successful coping and adaptation and incorporates assessment of these factors into an overall comprehensive plan of care.

The psychological impact of vision loss is reflected in the individual's coping and adaptation strategies. Coping refers to the cognitive, emotional, and behavioral responses made when confronted with an internally or externally created stressor. Adaptation, on the other hand, refers to a range of behaviors that include coping, but also goal setting, problem solving, and other active attempts to maintain psychological equilibrium (Hooyman & Kiyak, 2002). Knowledge of mental processes and their effects on behavior are critical for the nurse in caring for visually impaired older adults. A review of selected psychological theories is presented. The implications of these theories for how individuals cope with difficult or stressful life circumstances, specifically vision loss, are emphasized. However, the nurse also recognizes that coping and adaptation to aging and other concomitant health conditions is an ongoing task of late life development. Knowledge of these theories can assist the nurse in assessing, planning, and implementing effective care for visually impaired older adults.

Few would argue that age-related vision loss is a major stressor or life event that places significant demands on the older adult to satisfactorily cope and adapt. However, not everyone perceives this stressor in the same way. Psychological theories and research evidence suggest that certain characteristics are important in determining how older adults will respond to this major life event.

Some have suggested that, along with health and cognitive functioning, personality characteristics can influence coping (Hooyman & Kiyak, 2002). Costa and McCrae (1986) examined five broad domains of adjectives to characterize personality—neuroticism, extraversion, openness, agreeableness, and conscientiousness. They noted that these personality traits change little with age, although adulthood is a period of dynamic growth (Costa & McCrae, 1994). Research has been conducted that examined how these personality traits relate to adaptation to visual decline. Individuals who scored high on neuroticism (worry, temperamental, self-pity, self-conscious, emotional, and vulnerable) were more prone to experiencing negative consequences of physical stressors related to sensory declines. Those who had strong personality traits of extraversion (preference for social versus solitary activity; adjectives included affectionate, joiner, talkative, active, fun-loving, passionate) and openness (the degree to which an individual seeks new experiences and enjoys exploring unfamiliar environments; adjectives used included imaginative, creative, original, prefers variety, curious, liberal) were associated with positive emotional states. Jang and colleagues (2003) proposed that individuals with high levels of extraversion and openness would be more adaptive in responding to visual decline.

Jang et al. (2003) examined the significance of vision and hearing on physical, social and emotional functioning among older adults, along with the role of personality traits and social resources. Using a sample of 425 community-dwelling older adults (mean age: 72.2), the researchers found that vision loss was a significant factor for disability. Individuals with poorer vision were more likely to be older and had greater disability and higher levels of depressive symptoms. The association between sensory performance and depressive symptoms (using the Geriatric Depression Scale—Short Form) was not significant in multivariate analyses. However, the results did indicate that those with lower levels of neuroticism, higher levels of extraversion, and greater satisfaction with social support were less likely to be depressed. The authors conclude that these personality attributes might provide resilience against depressive symptoms and thus enable adjustment to sensory changes, including vision loss. Counseling and support could enable older adults with more neuroticism to gain insight into their behavior and could foster opportunities to enhance access to and use of social supports and visual rehabilitation interventions (Jang et al.).

Coping with vision loss is also influenced by the individual's cognitive appraisal of the stressor and subsequent reaction. Lazarus and Folkman (1984) introduced the concept of cognitive appraisal of significance and meaning as critical in determining one's response to stress. Cognitive appraisal is the way in which a person perceives the significance of an encounter or event for his or her well-being. Persons who perceive a particular situation as a challenge (positive stressor, which can offer a potential for growth) cope differently than those who view it as a threat (negative stressor, which threatens harm to the individual and evokes fear, anxiety, and anger). The challenge for nursing in caring for older visually impaired adults is to empower them to perceive visual impairment as a positive stressor or challenge that can be met with purposeful planning and access to and utilization of social and material resources.

The older adult's perception of the meaning of vision loss is also critical. This perception can affect one's self-concept, self-esteem, life satisfaction, successful aging, and quality of life. Individuals whose cognitive image of self (self-concept) and whose emotional assessment of the self (self-esteem) are based on a full-sighted identity will require a major adjustment. Whether the vision loss is of a sudden or gradual onset can also affect the perception of the stressor for older adults. The Holmes and Rahe (1967) Social Readjustment Rating Scale (SRRS), which measures major life-change units, would rank sudden vision loss sixth (as an example of personal injury or illness) among its 43 life-event stressors that could evoke significant physiological and psychological impact on individuals. A gradual onset in vision change might, on the other hand, contribute chronic daily hassles which, some suggest, can result in feelings of loneliness, lack of energy, regrets over past decisions, and concerns about one's current situation (Hooyman & Kiyak, 2002). Programs and services aimed at promoting visual rehabilitation, maximizing functional independence, and enhancing social supports are needed to counteract the major life disruption and chronic daily hassles posed by the vision loss.

Lawton (1982) introduced the person–environment fit model, which emphasizes the key role that the individual and environment have on one another. This is especially so for older adults experiencing vision loss. Older adults possess personal competencies that assist them in dealing with the environment. These competencies are ego strength, level of motor skills, individual biologic health, and cognitive and sensory–perceptual capacities (Lueckenotte, 2000). With age, and certainly with age-related vision loss, changes in these competencies affect the older person's ability to interrelate with the environment. Using Lawton's model, nurses could be instrumental in helping older adults to enhance their competence. Heyl and Wahl (2001), using the environmental press model, evaluated psychosocial adaptation to age-related vision loss among older visually impaired and older sighted individuals over a 6-year time period. Their findings stress the need to provide psychosocial intervention and rehabilitation at the earliest possible time to prevent unnecessary dependence and the loss of autonomy in the future. Older adults should be encouraged to utilize unrecognized potential, noting their increased self-esteem when handling stress effectively and active mastery when taking control over and satisfactorily responding to environmental demands (Lawton, 1982).

Baltes's (1987) selective optimization compensation model of successful aging posits that individuals develop certain strategies to manage the losses of function that occur over time. Using vision loss as an example, successful aging can occur when the three interacting elements, selection (restricting one's life to fewer domains of functioning because of age-related vision loss), optimization (whereby persons engage in behaviors to enrich their lives), and compensation (in which older adults compensate for their vision loss by developing suitable, alternative adaptations), are employed (Lueckenotte, 2000). Achievement of successful aging, defined by Rowe and Kahn (1998) as "absence of disease and disability, maintaining high cognitive and physical function, and active engagement with life" (p. 39), is possible despite visual impairments. Older adults can select those specific domains of functioning they wish to maximize. They can optimize their remaining abilities instead of dwelling on the actual impairment. They can compensate for the vision loss through the use of education, community resources, counseling and support, and visual rehabilitation programs.

Experience of Vision Loss

Although psychological theories can be helpful in understanding what to assess, how to intervene, and what to evaluate in caring for visually impaired older adults, the actual lived experience of older adults with these vision changes is equally important for nurses to understand. Among the reported factors correlated with vision loss in older adults have been psychological distress, low morale, and depression; reduced self-worth, diminished emotional security and quality of life and well-being; and altered functional status (Barzargan, Baker, & Bazargan, 2001). Moore and Miller (2003) used a phenomenological approach to investigate the experience of severe visual impairment in eight older men with macular degeneration. Six central themes emerged: "(1) older men's lives were circumscribed by what they could and could not see and could and could not do, (2) cherishing of independence, (3) creation of strategies, (4) acknowledgement of the progression of visual impairment, (5) confrontation of uncertainties, skepticism, and fears about their diagnosis and treatment, and (6) persistence with hope and optimism" (Moore & Miller, p. 10). Health histories and assessments should incorporate information related to each of these themes, along with needed education and effective communication.

The majority of older adults who experience late-life onset of vision change still have some usable vision (Ryan, Anas, Beamer, & Bajorek, 2003). Some have compared the loss of vision as similar to the feelings of losing a loved one, in that the grieving process in many ways applies to the loss of vision (Kelch, 2000). The attitudes and beliefs of the older adult about blindness or about people with disabilities can affect this grieving process, as can an individual's prior response to stress. Both qualitative and quantitative research methodologies have been used to examine the experience of vision loss.

In a qualitative study, Brennan and colleagues (2001) utilized narrative data from three previous quantitative studies to address the strategies developed by visually impaired elders to cope with vision loss. The typology of coding for coping strategies was categorized into behavioral, psychological, and social domains. Examples of the behavioral strategies reported by participants include overt, observable actions, such as seeking and using optical and adaptive devices, voluntarily reducing or ceasing driving, and acting more cautiously. Psychological coping strategies included emotions and cognitions, such as expressing anger toward oneself or others and recognizing that others have similar problems. Social coping involved the utilization of informal social networks, support groups or counseling sessions, and formal care providers.

For the psychological coping strategies, the researchers developed eight different families of coping strategies: "relies on personal resources, engages situation, accepts vision impairment, uses cognitive refocusing, avoids negative thoughts or feelings, expresses negative thoughts or feelings, makes attributions of cause, and expresses hope" (Brennan et al., 2001, p. 72). The researchers concluded that participants recognized a need to balance cultural and personal norms of independence against those functional losses resulting from age-related vision impairment. Additionally, the importance of engaging social support in assisting the older person to adapt was noted. Key for the participants was that different strategies across all three domains—behavioral, psychological, and social—were utilized, suggesting that older visually impaired adults attempt to adapt using a variety of different methods.

Age-related vision loss can also result in an older adult's use of preexisting as well as novel coping strategies in adaptation. Brennan and Cardinali (2000) note that individuals experiencing vision loss may test novel coping strategies when preexisting strategies fail. They note that vision loss disrupts patterns of behavior, the psychological domains of body image and self-concept, and social interaction. Identifying how older adults use coping strategies, both preexisting and novel, was the purpose of their study.

In this study, Brennan and Cardinali (2000) used both qualitative and quantitative techniques. The qualitative analysis was used for the initial identification of self-reported coping strategies and the subsequent classification of each as novel or preexisting. Coping strategies were coded as preexisting if the strategy was used prior to the onset of vision loss, and novel strategies were categorized as such if the strategy was implemented in direct response to the vision impairment or was recently adopted. The results indicate that preexisting coping strategies were most likely to be found in the psychological domain (56%; $n = 331$), followed by the social domain (30%; $n = 181$) and the behavioral domain (14%; $n = 84$). Novel coping strategies, on the other hand, were most likely in the behavioral domain (45%; $n = 729$), followed by the psychological (34%; $n = 511$) and social (17%; $n = 249$) domains (Brennan & Cardinali). Examples of novel coping strategies within the behavioral domain included seeking services to learn skills and seeking or using adaptive or optical devices. Novel psychological strategies included acceptance of vision loss or greater emphasis on abilities rather than on limitations. Lee and Brennan (2003) described coping strategies in the social domain as activating formal services and seeking informal advice, emotional support, and visual information help; attending group meetings/support groups; relying on family, friends; talking over problems and learning from others with visual impairment; or choosing to withdraw socially.

The quantitative component of the study used the Adaptation to Age-Related Vision Loss Scale (Horowitz & Reinhardt, 1998) (Table 7.2) and the Center for Epidemiological Studies Depression scale (CES-D) (Radloff, 1977).

TABLE 7.2 Adaptation to Vision Loss (AVL) Scale

Test administrator should read the following: NEXT, I WILL READ SOME STATEMENTS THAT HAVE BEEN MADE ABOUT VISION IMPAIRMENT. SOME PEOPLE MAY AGREE WITH THESE STATEMENTS AND OTHERS MAY DISAGREE.

AS I READ EACH STATEMENT, PLEASE TELL ME WHETHER YOU STRONGLY AGREE, SOMEWHAT AGREE, SOMEWHAT DISAGREE, OR STRONGLY DISAGREE.

	Strongly Agree	Somewhat Agree	Somewhat Disagree	Strongly Disagree	D/K
1. Because of my vision loss, I feel like I can never really do things for myself.	0	1	2	3	9
2. Most service available to visually impaired persons are useless in really helping them with their problems.	0	1	2	3	9
3. I can still do many of the things I love, it just takes me longer because of my vision impairment.	3	2	1	0	9
4. Visual impairment is the cause of all my problems.	0	1	2	3	9
5. Some people in the family act as though the visually impaired person is a burden to them.	0	1	2	3	9
6. A visually impaired person can never really be happy.	0	1	2	3	9
7. Because of my trouble seeing, I am afraid that people will take advantage of me.	0	1	2	3	9
8. By learning new ways of doing things (that compensate for vision loss), a visually impaired person has a chance to be more independent.	3	2	1	0	9
9. Visually impaired persons cannot afford to talk back or argue with family and friends.	0	1	2	3	9
10. People should not expect too much from visually impaired persons.	0	1	2	3	9
11. People who experience vision loss late in life will never be able to learn how to get around without bumping into things.	0	1	2	3	9
12. It is too hard for older people to learn new ways of doing things (that compensate for vision loss) if they become visually impaired.	0	1	2	3	9
13. Visually impaired people might as well accept the fact that vision impairment makes people pretty helpless.	0	1	2	3	9

(Continued)

117

TABLE 7.2 Adaptation to Vision Loss (AVL) Scale (cont.)

	Strongly Agree	Somewhat Agree	Somewhat Disagree	Strongly Disagree	D/K
14. It is degrading for visually impaired persons to depend so much on family and friends.	0	1	2	3	9
15. Although the circumstances of my life have been changed, I am still the same person I was before my vision impairment.	3	2	1	0	9
16. Sighted people generally dislike being with visually impaired people (because of their vision problems).	0	1	2	3	9
17. Sighted people expect visually impaired persons to do things that are impossible.	0	1	2	3	9
18. Visually impaired people have to depend on sighted people to do most of the things they did for themselves.	0	1	2	3	9
19. Losing one's sight means losing one's self.	0	1	2	3	9
20. People with vision problems are uncomfortable making new friends because they cannot always see people's faces clearly.	0	1	2	3	9
21. I feel comfortable asking my family and friends for help with things I can no longer do because of my vision loss.	3	2	1	0	9
22. When a person become visually impaired, sighted friends don't understand him or her as they did before.	0	1	2	3	9
23. It is better for a person with vision problems to let other people do things for them.	0	1	2	3	9
24. There are worse things that can happen to a person than losing vision.	3	2	1	0	9

Source: Retrieved October 23, 2004, from http//www.visionconnection.org/Content/Research/PsychosocialandEvaluationResearch/. From Horowitz, A., & Reinhardt, J. P. (1998). Psychological adjustment to vision impairment among the elderly: Development of the Adaptation to Age-Related Vision Loss (AVL) Scale. *Journal of Visual Impairment and Blindness, 92,* 30–41. Reprinted with permission from Lighthouse International.

Results revealed that those using a greater number of novel social coping strategies demonstrated a significant, positive correlation with Adaptation to Age-Related Vision Loss scores suggesting better adaptation. The use of novel coping at the 2-year follow-up was also associated with better adjustment to vision loss and fewer depressive symptoms. The authors suggest that novel coping strategies may serve to enhance, rather than replace, habitual ways of coping. Targeting interventions for older adults with vision impairment should address the need to bolster preexisting coping strategies and offer alternative approaches to enhance adaptation.

Reinhardt and Benn (2000) studied the role of personal and social resources in elders' adaptation to chronic vision loss. They found better adaptation "associated with higher income adequacy, less functional disability, greater use of acceptance coping and less use of wishfulness coping, and instrumental and affective support received from one's family" (p. 653). The authors suggest encouraging the use of acceptance coping in older adults to enable better adaptation to vision loss.

Many nursing diagnoses have relevance for understanding the psychological impact of vision loss on older adults. Nursing diagnosis is "A clinical judgment about individual, family, or community responses to actual or potential health problems/life processes. A nursing diagnosis provides the basis for selection of nursing interventions to achieve outcomes for which the nurse is accountable" (NANDA, 2003, p. 263). Through the University of Iowa College of Nursing and NANDA, a team of nurse researchers uses concept analyses, expert validation, and other research methodologies to establish these diagnoses. Among diagnoses with relevance to vision loss are those from the Perceiving Pattern. "This pattern involves the reception of information; to apprehend what is not open or present to observation. The nursing diagnoses include Disturbance in Body Image, Self-Esteem, or Personal Identity; Sensory/Perceptual Alterations; Hopelessness; and Powerlessness. The major concepts are self-concept, sensory responses, and meaningfulness" (Craven & Hirnle, 2000, p. 183).

However, other nursing diagnoses are also impacted by vision loss in older adults. Examples of nursing diagnoses that should be considered in the assessment and care planning for the older adult with vision loss are: Impaired Adjustment, Ineffective Coping, Risk for Loneliness, Risk for Powerlessness, Ineffective Role Performance, Self-Care Deficit, Situational Low Self-Esteem, Impaired Social Interaction, Impaired Home Maintenance, Fear, Anxiety, Altered Thought Processes, Social Isolation, and Spiritual Distress.

Spirituality has been shown to impact psychological adaptation to vision loss (Brennan, 2002), with high levels of spirituality and religiousness leading to improved outcomes to stressful life events. Using a single-group, correlational design, Brennan tested the relationships among exogenous variables (sociodemographics, life experience, and vision status), mediating variables (spirituality, religiousness, and social support), and psychosocial development as an outcome measure. Results suggested that life-event stress might serve to further personal growth on the part of the individual. Spirituality was found to be a strong predictor of psychosocial development and a buffer to negative life experiences. This effect was strongest when individuals characterized their vision impairment as having both a negative impact and not being under their control (Brennan).

The functional losses that may accompany vision loss demand a psychological response from the older adult. Vision impairment and functioning among community-dwelling older Americans were examined by Crews and Campbell (2004). The findings revealed that older individuals with vision impairment were more likely to report difficulty walking than people without sensory problems (39.0% vs. 17.8%), and more likely to report difficulty getting outside than people without sensory problems (25.1% vs. 9.3%). The same group of older adults self-reported being more likely to have difficulty getting into and out of a bed or chair (19.4% vs. 8.0%), more likely to report difficulty managing medication (10.8% vs. 3.7%), and more likely to report difficulty preparing meals (19.2% vs. 6.3%). This decline in functional ability can have a negative social and psychological impact on older adults with vision loss.

Brennan, Horowtiz, and Su (2002) reported on data from four waves of the Longitudinal Study on Aging (LSOA), which examined the consequences of dual sensory impairment among U.S. adults 70 years and older ($n = 5,151$). Although dual (vision and hearing) sensory impairment was associated with lower functional ability, more help received with activities of daily living (ADL) and instrumental activities of daily living (IADL) tasks, and difficulties with physical functioning, the authors note that the negative effects are largely due to the vision loss. Specifically, offering assistance for those activities required for independence in everyday living—self-care, communication, and mobility skills—could be helpful to maintain psychological well-being and social involvement in the community.

In a study by Bazargan, Baker, and Bazargan (2001), the impact of dual sensory impairments and subjective well-being among 998 older African-American persons was examined using bivariate and multivariate techniques. The findings revealed that lower psychological well-being was found among older African American persons who "were female, with poor vision, more financial problems, a higher level of cognitive deficit, more stressful life events, lower levels of health status, and more limitations in daily activities due to chronic illnesses" (Bazargan et al., p. P273). The finding of a lower level of psychological well-being was greater for persons with visual impairments, even when functional limitation, perceived health status, and cognition were controlled for. These findings suggest that visual impairment may have a significantly greater burden among older African Americans "compared with prevalence rates reported for the general aged American (i.e., predominantly White) population" (Bazargan et al., p. P274), when sociodemographic variables are taken into consideration.

Given the importance older adults place on functional independence, it is clear that the psychological impact of dealing with functional limitations places an added burden on the visually impaired elder. Verbrugge and Jette (1994) offer a model for understanding how psychological factors and other internal resources of individuals can impact the pathway of pathology to disability. They define disability as difficulty doing activities in any life domain due to a health or physical problem. Disability is not a personal characteristic but a gap between personal capability and environmental demands (Verbruge & Jette). The Disablement Model suggests that reducing the environmental demands or increasing the capabilities of the individual can interrupt this disability pathway. Additionally, they point to the importance of such psychological attributes as mastery and self-efficacy, life satisfaction, and locus of control in altering this pathway, even after controlling for functional limitations. Social support is another resource that can alter the trajectory to disability. Thus, emphasizing an individual's capability through activity accommodation, environmental modification, psychological coping, and external supports can aid the visually impaired older adult.

In defining disability and functioning, the WHO describes the existing medical and social models in use. The medical model "views disability as a problem of the person, directly caused by disease, trauma or other health condition, which requires medical care provided in the form of individual treatment by professionals. Management of the disability is aimed at cure or the individual's adjustment and behavior change" (WHO, 2001, p. 20). Social models, on the other hand, see the issue mainly as a socially created problem where disability is not an attribute of the individual but a complex set of factors created by the social environment. In the social model, society must make the environmental modifications necessary for the full participation of persons with disabilities in all areas of social life. The International Classification of Functioning (WHO) integrates both of these models and uses a biopsychosocial approach. Thus, disablement is conceptualized along three dimensions: impairment, activities, and participation. "Impairments are problems in body function or structure such as a significant deviation or loss; activity is the execution of a task or action by an individual; participation is involvement in a life situation" (WHO, p. 10). The nurse should incorporate assessment of the internal and external variables that impact a visually impaired elder's coping and adaptation in establishing plans of care.

One functional loss that has a tremendous impact on visually impaired older adults is reading. Given that the most common age-related eye disease is macular degeneration, this impairment will result in difficulty seeing print. The difficulty in reading can affect leisure activities (playing cards, reading books, and writing letters) and functional independence (shopping and handling finances) (Ryan et al., 2003). Ryan et al. explored reading in older adults with visual impairment, using a convenience sample of late-onset, moderately and severely, visually impaired older adults. Eighteen women and eight men, ranging in age from 65 to 93, were recruited from ophthalmologic practices to participate in qualitative interviews.

The purpose of the study was to clarify the role of reading for leisure and how participants dealt with reading required for instrumental activities of daily living. The participants reported that reading was just as important after as it was before their vision loss, although there was a decline in use of newspapers and magazines. Almost 60% used talking books, whereas 25% used computer technology for reading print. The participants identified that the demands of small print, dials, and currency affected their performance in reading and instrumental activities of daily living. Particularly, reading expiration dates, labels, and recipes affected meal preparation. Numbers on telephones and locating address book information impacted telephone use. Reading involving checks, deposit slips, bills and receipts, and ATM machine use made dealing with finances difficult. Travel was problematic, as it related to signs, bus schedules, maps, and various electronic schedule boards. Appliance use, instruction manuals or warranties, labels on cleaning products, and dials or buttons on washing machines and dryers offered challenges in the laundry area. Both medication use and shopping were affected by labels on bottles, medication instructions, and reading of prices and expiration dates (Ryan et al., 2003).

Using the Baltes (1987) framework of selection, optimization, and compensation, Ryan et al. (2003) reported on the effective strategies employed by participants. The person-oriented strategies involved selection and optimization, whereas the environment-oriented strategies dealt with compensation. Examples provided by participants about the person-oriented strategies used included selecting realistic goals and relying on memory and new learning to adapt to age-related vision changes. Environment-oriented strategies offered by the participants were the use of optical devices and reliance on others to maintain functional independence. Offering of these varied strategies by the nurse may prove helpful in enabling older adults to adjust to age-related vision loss.

SOCIAL IMPACT OF AGE-RELATED VISION LOSS

Social role participation and social interaction are key for positive adjustment in old age. For older adults experiencing a vision loss, both may be affected, and these changes can severely limit opportunities for sustaining one's self-concept and self-esteem. As Table 7.1 (WHO, 2001) notes, contextual factors in the environment can facilitate adaptation of the older adult to visual impairment by addressing the impact of the physical, social, and attitudinal world in maintaining the individual's functional integrity and activity participation. Key among the successful interventions for visually impaired older adults would be vocational rehabilitation, visual rehabilitation, optical technologies, community resources (transportation, housing, income adequacy, services, and programs and public policies targeted to the visually impaired), and adequate and satisfying social networks.

Role losses that may be experienced by visually impaired older adults can further limit functional independence. These losses may relate to being able to maintain independent living environments, employment and volunteering opportunities, and ready access to transportation that includes driving an automobile. Leisure role activities, such as hobbies, interests, and recreation, are also impacted. Each of these roles is strongly associated with perceived functional independence and quality of life.

Driving is a measure of self-reliance for many older adults. As such, its limitation or cessation can have serious consequences. Rosenblum and Corn (2002) evaluated the experiences of older adults who stopped driving because of their visual impairments. Using qualitative data from focus groups and two in-depth interviews with older adult nondrivers, the researchers drafted an instrument that sought information about how older adults chose to stop driving and whether residence or relationships with family and friends changed as a result. The survey was administered in one-to-one in-person or telephone interviews with 162 individuals recruited through a variety of means. Nearly 70% of the participants themselves decided to give up driving because they reported not being able to see well enough to continue driving; another 13.6% were told by an ophthalmologist that it was time to drop driving. The remaining responses offered by participants were: told by another physician; their children or other family members; had an accident and decided to stop; had licenses revoked by state department of motor vehicles; or had other experiences that led them to stop, such as an instant loss of vision (Rosenblum & Corn).

As a result of driving cessation, older adults reported seeking assistance to travel to a destination. Thirty percent traveled without assistance in unfamiliar places, whereas 38% needed some assistance and 13% used a sighted guide.

An additional 18.5% reported seldom traveling so they had little need to go to unfamiliar places. For those who required assistance, 47.5% mentioned sighted persons accompanying them, with another 46% mentioning white canes.

Activity change due to driving cessation resulted in 67.3% of the sample having to make changes in their lifestyle. These included 27.8% who changed their residence, 33.8% who stopped working, and 34% who stopped doing volunteer work. Those reporting that they stopped working did so because of their inability to drive, not because of the functional problems related to poor vision (Rosenblum & Corn, 2002). Thus, work and leisure role losses could be counteracted by nurses who provide the support or education needed to access needed transportation services. Helpful Web sites for accessing information about advocacy for better access, including financing, are available from: http://www.visionconnection.org (Vision Connection), http://www.nei.nih.gov (National Eye Institute of the U.S. NIH), and http://www.lighthouse.org/advocacy/legislation_vision_services.htm (Lighthouse International).

Leisure roles and activity participation are important for the social and psychological well-being and life satisfaction of older adults. In general, leisure activities, including social and home-based activities, may be increasingly important during the retirement years. Visual impairment will require environmental modifications so that continued involvement in valued leisure time activities, and the satisfaction derived from these, can be maintained. However, for those activities that require the greatest visual ability, disengagement may be an adaptive strategy (Burmedi, Becker, Heyl, Wahl, & Himmelsbach, 2002a). Burmedi et al.'s review of the research on the behavioral consequences of age-related low vision suggests that Baltes's (1987) selection, optimization, and compensation model may apply. Thus, those life domains of greatest importance (social interaction, for instance) may be selected and optimized, while leisure activities requiring visual acuity are reduced and greater reliance is placed on other resources (i.e., relationships) for compensation (Burmedi et al.). For example, for individuals who enjoyed journal writing but now have difficulty reading or writing due to visual impairments, the use of an audio diary could substitute for this valued activity (Papadopoulos & Scanlon, 2002).

In a qualitative research study, two case studies were presented to explore how older adults' visual impairments impacted on their adaptation to enable them to engage in community- and home-based leisure activities (Stevens-Ratchford & Krause, 2004). Key among the leisure role changes reported by both participants was the loss of their ability to drive. This loss resulted in the "end of spontaneity and independence in freely choosing and participating in community-based activities" (Stevens-Ratchford & Krause, pp. 19–20).

Environmental modifications made to adapt to the discrepancy between the abilities and the demands of the environment included use of optical and nonoptical (talking clocks) devices, maintaining order and structure in the home, and strategic organization (one participant's granddaughter organized a collection of videotapes in alphabetical order to help in finding a desired movie). Both participants expressed their view that maintaining involvement in leisure activities was key to their sense of well-being. Particularly important was the notion of social engagement with life—whether through home- or community-based activities. Both participants had made home modifications, but neither was willing to make any further changes, as each felt supported by the familiarity of their home.

Social interaction, in the form of relationships (which can also include formal religious activity participation) and availability and satisfaction with social networks, is a variable that is believed crucial for well-being in older visually impaired adults. In a 20-year extensive review of literature on the emotional and social consequences of age-related low vision, it was found that: "Social support seems to be an effective buffer against the negative effects associated with vision loss, like depression or a decrease in life satisfaction, and to enhance adaptation to vision loss" (Burmedi, Becker, Heyl, Wahl, & Himmelsbach, 2002b, p. 64). And yet, environments that accommodate the special needs associated with visual loss to maintain social roles and enhance social interactions are often lacking.

Social support from family and friends has been recognized as a key determinant of well-being among older adults. For those older adults with vision loss, the value of social support assumes an even greater importance. Horowitz, Reinhardt, Brennan and Cantor (1997) found that those who had contact with someone outside the family who experienced a vision loss, those with greater knowledge about vision loss and aging, self-reported higher education, and higher income were found to have a more positive attitude about vision loss. Others have suggested that understanding of an older adult's adaptation to low vision must include attention to relationship patterns (Travis et al., 2003). Travis et al. studied 25 participants recruited from a low-vision clinic and found that 48% were accompanied by family members (most often adult children) and friends. Thus, family members' and friends' involvement in and understanding of the process and outcome of vision rehabilitation services could contribute to the elder's adaptation. Heine and Browning (2002) also note the importance of a visually impaired person's attitude toward social relationships with family members, friends, and other members of society in the statement, "Balance lies in neither rejecting assistance nor excessively depending on others" (p. 769).

Another study on social support and loneliness in older visually impaired adults found that those satisfied with their social support network reported less loneliness than those who were not (Barron, Foxall, VonDollen, Jones, & Shull, 1994). Importantly, these researchers found that the satisfaction with the support received, not the size of the network, was found to predict less loneliness. Reinhardt (1996) found supportive friendships and family relationships, less functional disability, and higher education to be positive predictors of adaptation to vision loss.

The key importance of social support was identified as well in a study that investigated factors associated with better initial adaptation to visual impairment. Higher quality of the relationship with the closest family member and feeling that family members understand one's limitations were related to adaptation (Horowitz, Reinhardt, McInerny, Balistreri, & Serapio, 1994). In another study, the relationship between marital status, social support, and loneliness in 87 visually impaired older adults was examined (Barron et al., 1994). Their results revealed that marital status did not predict either the degree of loneliness or social support network size or satisfaction. Network size, however, was higher for nonlonely than for lonely respondents. Dissatisfaction with the caring network was the second largest predictor of loneliness (Barron et al., 1994). The authors propose that nurses intervene for visually impaired older adults by mutually strategizing ways to increase social network size and by encouraging the older adult to communicate their expectations to network members. Such proactive behaviors might prevent or alleviate loneliness and increase well-being and adaptation to the vision loss.

SUCCESSFUL AGING AND QUALITY OF LIFE WITH VISION LOSS

Vision impairment is a common and serious chronic condition experienced by an increasing number of older adults that results in functional impairment. Given that some have suggested successful aging encompasses cognitive ability, functional independence, and engagement with others (Rowe & Kahn, 1998), nurses might ask whether the goal of successful aging with vision impairment is possible. Research suggests that it not only is possible, but also it is actively occurring. Strawbridge, Wallhagen, and Cohen (2002) evaluated the Rowe and Kahn model of successful aging in their study of 867 Alameda County Study participants, ages 65 to 99 with various chronic conditions and functional impairments, by comparing participant self-ratings of successful aging to the researchers' ratings based on the Rowe and Kahn criteria. They found that 50.3% of participants self-rated themselves as aging successfully compared to 18.8% when researchers used the Rowe and Kahn criteria exclusively.

Learning to live with oneself as one's vision changes, and adapting to this vision loss by learning a way to live according to a particular set of values, is a necessary prerequisite for the quality-of-life goal of older visually impaired adults. Personality attributes, cognitive appraisal of the stressor of vision loss, recognition of the person-oriented and environment-oriented contextual factors that impact activity limitation, emphasizing ability versus disability, and engaging previous and new coping strategies all impact on the psychological well-being of older adults with vision loss.

Social roles and social interaction remain critical elements in adapting to age, and especially so when vision loss is a part of this aging process. Support groups can offer many benefits for the visually impaired elder, including education, insights, and emotional assistance. Environments that foster independence for the older adult, while recognizing the important need for interdependence as well, are necessary to achieve social well-being. Knowledge of available community resources and supports can further enhance this adaptation process.

REFERENCES

Baltes, P. B. (1987). *Life-span development and behavior*. Volume 7. Hillsdale, NJ: Lawrence Erlbaum Associates.

Barron, C. R., Foxall, M. J., VonDollen, K., Jones, P. A. & Shull, K. A. (1994). Marital status, social support, and loneliness in visually impaired elderly people. *Journal of Advanced Nursing, 19*(2), 272–280.

Bazargan, M., Baker, R. S., & Bazargan, S. H. (2001). Sensory impairments and subjective well-being among aged African American persons. *Journal of Gerontology: Psychological Sciences, 56B*(5), P268–P278.

Brennan, M. (2002). Spirituality and psychosocial development in middle-age and older adults with vision loss. *Journal of Adult Development, 9*(1), 31–46.

Brennan, M. (2003). Impairment in both vision and hearing among older adults: Prevalence and impact on quality of life. *Generations, 27*, 52–56.

Brennan, M., & Cardinali, G. (2000). The use of preexisting and novel coping strategies in adapting to age-related vision loss. *The Gerontologist, 40*(3), 327–334.

Brennan, M., Horowitz, A., Reinhardt, J. P., Cimarolli, V., Benn, D. T., & Leonard, R. (2001). In their own words: Strategies developed by visually impaired elders to cope with vision loss. *Journal of Gerontological Social Work, 35*(1), 63–85.

Brennan, M., Horowitz, A., & Su, Y-P. (November 2002). *The widespread consequences of dual sensory loss among older U.S. Adults*. In I. Lissman & K. Boerner (Chairs), *Consequences of sensory loss in old age*. Symposium conducted at the

Annual Scientific Meeting of the Gerontological Society of America. Boston, MA.

Burmedi, D., Becker, S., Heyl, V., Wahl, H. W., & Himmelsbach, I. (2002a). Behavioral consequences of age-related low vision: A narrative review. *Visual Impairmen Research*, 4(1), 15–45.

Burmedi, D., Becker, S., Heyl, V., Wahl, H. W., & Himmelsbach, I. (2002b). Emotional and social consequences of age-related low vision: A narrative review. *Visual Impairment Research*, 4(1), 47–71.

Campbell, V. C., Crews, J. E., Moriarty, D. G., Zack, M. M., & Blackman, D. K. (1999). Surveillance for sensory impairment, activity limitation, and health-related quality of life among older adults. United States, 1993–1997. *Surveillance Summaries*, 48(SS08), 131–156.

Costa, P. T., & McCrae, R. R. (1986). Personality stability and its implications for clinical psychology. *Clinical Psychology Review*, 6(5), 407–423.

Costa, P. T., & McCrae, R. R. (1994). Personality and aging. In W. R. Hazzard, E. L. Bierman, J. P. Blass, W. H. Ettinger, & J. B. Halter (Eds.), *Principles of geriatric medicine and gerontology* (3rd ed.; pp. 107–113). New York: McGraw-Hill.

Craven, R. F., & Hirnle, C. J. (2000). *Fundamentals of nursing: Human health and function* (3rd ed.). Philadelphia: Lippincott.

Crews, J. E., & Campbell, V. A. (2004). Vision impairment and hearing loss among community-dwelling older Americans: Implications for health and functioning. *American Journal of Public Health*, 94(5), 823–829.

Heine, C., & Browning, C. J. (2002). Communication and psychosocial consequences of sensory loss in older adults: Overview and rehabilitation directions. *Disability and Rehabilitation*, 24(15), 763–773.

Heyl, V., & Wahl, H. W. (2001). Psychosocial adaptation to age-related vision loss: A six-year perspective. *Journal of Visual Impairment & Blindness*, 95(12), 739–748.

Holmes, T. H., & Rahe, R. (1967). The social readjustment rating scale. *Journal of Psychosomatic Research*, 11(2), 213–218.

Hooyman, N. R., & Kiyak, H. A. (2002). *Social gerontology: A multidisciplinary perspective* (6th ed.). Boston: Allyn & Bacon.

Horowitz, A., & Reinhardt, J. P. (1998). Psychosocial adjustment to vision impairment among the elderly: Development of the Adaptation to Age-Related Vision Loss Scale. *Journal of Visual Impairment and Blindness*, 92(1), 30–44. Retrieved July 10, 2004, from EBSCOhost.

Horowitz, A., Reinhardt, J. P., Brennan, M., & Cantor, M. (1997). *Aging and vision loss: Experiences, attitudes, and knowledge of older Americans*. New York: Arlene R. Gordon Research Institute, Lighthouse International.

Horowitz, A., Reinhardt, J. P., McInerny, R., Balistreri, E., & Serapio, J.G. (1994). *Age-related vision loss. Factors associated with adaptation to chronic impairment over time*. New York: The Lighthouse, Inc.

Jang, Y., Mortimer, J. A., Haley, W. E., Small, B. J., Chisolm, T. E. H., & Graves, A. B. (2003). The role of vision and hearing in physical, social, and emotional functioning among older adults. *Research on Aging*, 25(2), 172–192.

Kelch, J. (2000). Coping with the dark side: The psychosocial implications of sudden vision loss due to trauma. *Topics in Emergency Medicine, 22*(4), 9–13.

Lawton, M. P. (1982). Competence, environmental press, and the adaptation of older people (pp. 33–59). In M. P. Lawton, P. G. Windley, & T. O. Byerts (Eds.), *Aging and the environment: Theoretical approaches.* New York: Springer.

Lazarus, R. S., & Folkman, S. (1984). *Stress, appraisal, and coping.* New York: Springer.

Lee, E. K.O., & Brennan, M. (2003). I am the fighter until the last moment: The relation of race/ethnicity and education to self-reported coping strategies among older adults with vision impairment. *Journal of Social Work in Disability and Rehabilitation, 2*(4), 3–28.

Lueckenotte, A. G. (2000). *Gerontologic nursing* (2nd ed.). St. Louis: C.V. Mosby.

Moore, L. W., & Miller, J. (2003). Older men's experiences of living with severe visual impairment. *Journal of Advanced Nursing, 43*(1), 10–18.

NANDA. (2003). *NANDA Nursing diagnoses: Definitions & classification 2003–2004.* Philadelphia: NANDA International.

Papadopoulos, I., & Scanlon, K. (2002). The use of audio diaries in a study with visually impaired people. *Journal of Visual Impairment & Blindness, 96*(6), 456–459.

Pleis, J. R., & Coles, R. (2003). *Summary health statistics for U.S. adults: National Health Interview Survey, 1999.* Vital and Health Statistics, Series 10, Number 212. Hyattsville, MD: National Center for Health Statistics, DHHS Publication No. (PHS) 2003–1540.

Radloff, L. S. (1977). The CES-D scale: A self-report depression scale for research in the general population. *Applied Psychological Measurement, 1,* 385–401.

Reinhardt, J. P. (1996). The importance of friendship and family support in adaptation to chronic vision impairment. *Journal of Gerontology: Psychological Sciences, 51B*(5), P268–P278.

Reinhardt, J. P., & Benn, D. (2000). The role of personal and social resources in elders' adaptation to chronic vision loss. In C. Stuen, A. Arditi, A. Horowitz, M. A. Lang, B. Rosenthal, & K. R. Seidman (Eds.), *Vision rehabilitation: Assessment, intervention and outcomes* (pp. 650–654). Lisse, The Netherlands: Swets & Zeitlinger Publishers.

Rosenblum, L. P., & Corn, A. L. (2002). Experiences of older adults who stopped driving because of their visual impairments: Part 1. *Journal of Visual Impairment & Blindness, 96*(6), 389–398.

Rowe, J. W., & Kahn, R. L. (1998). *Successful aging.* New York: Pantheon Books.

Ryan, E. B., Anas, A. P., Beamer, M., & Bajorek, S. (2003). Coping with age-related vision loss in everyday reading activities. *Educational Gerontology, 29,* 37–54.

Stevens-Ratchford, R., & Krause, A. (2004). Visually impaired older adults and home-based leisure activities: The effects of person-environment congruence. *Journal of Visual Impairment & Blindness, 98*(1), 14–27.

Strawbridge, W. J., Wallhagen, M. I., & Cohen, R. D. (2002). Successful aging and well-being: Self-rated compared with Rowe and Kahn. *The Gerontologist, 42*(6), 727–733.

Travis, L. A., Lyness, J. M., Sterns, G. W., Kuchmek, M., Shielf, C. G., King, D. A., Sterns, S., & Northrup, L. (2003). Family and friends: A key aspect of older adults' adaptation to low vision? *Journal of Visual Impairment & Blindness, 97*(8), 489–492.

U.S. Department of Health and Human Services. (2001). *Healthy people 2010*. Washington, DC: U.S. Department of Health and Human Services. Retrieved July 7, 2004, from http://www.healthypeople.gov/Document/HTML/volume2/28Vision.htm

Verbrugge, L. M., & Jette, A. M. (1994). The disablement process. *Social Science and Medicine, 38*(1), 1–14.

World Health Organization. (2001). *International classification of functioning, disability and health*. Retrieved July 7, 2004, from http://www.WHO.int/classification/icf/intros/ICF-Eng-Intro.pdf

CHAPTER 8

Nursing Care of Older Adults With Age-Related Vision Loss

Pamela Z. Cacchione

Sensory impairment due to low vision greatly impacts the development of the nursing care plan for older adults. Nursing care for older adults with vision loss includes completing a comprehensive health assessment and planning, implementing, and evaluating nursing interventions for the purpose of achieving expected outcomes. Caring for older adults with low vision regardless of the setting should proceed using this framework, but must begin with a thorough assessment of the level of vision impairment. The heterogeneity of an older adult's response to vision impairment precludes a nurse from becoming complacent with vision assessments. Nurses cannot depend on self-report of visual impairment due to underreporting of symptoms. Studies have shown that older adults tend to underestimate their level of vision impairment. Questions about vision have a low sensitivity for detecting vision impairment when compared to formal acuity testing (Smeeth, 1998).

Visual function in older adults impacts their ability to care for themselves and may support or hamper nursing care. Vision is an essential part of everyday life, depended on constantly by people at all ages. Vision affects development, learning, communicating, working, and health and quality of life (National Institutes of Health, 2002). An older adult's ability to see impacts the ability to read instructions, negotiate their environment, and communicate effectively, and it is important in providing adequate self-care. Upon encountering a new older adult client, the nurse should complete a thorough assessment of the client's functional vision. An individualized vision assessment starts with obtaining a vision health history followed by completing the following assessments: visual acuity, near and distance vision, contrast sensitivity, and visual fields. With advanced education and training, nurses can complete comprehensive vision assessments, such as fundus exams using a pan ophthal-moscope, to evaluate the older individual's retina, macula, and optic nerve, all of which can be affected by the age-related changes and pathological conditions described in the preceding chapters.

Understanding the individual's level of functional vision is important in providing individualized nursing care, particularly patient teaching, medica-tion safety, and environmental safety. Visual impairment from most eye diseases and disorders can be reduced with early detection and treatment (National In-stitute of Health, 2002). Nurses have an important role in maintaining current sight and preventing blindness in older adults. Nurses should also assist older adults in adaptation to low vision, utilization of adaptive equipment, and use of visual devices such as lenses, magnification, and assistive technology. This can be accomplished by assessing the older adult, monitoring vision, and providing nursing care to older adults with chronic or acute eye conditions.

VISION ASSESSMENT

Vision Health History

A vision assessment begins with a comprehensive history of the older adult's vision in order to gather health history information, as well as an assessment into his or her awareness of visual functioning or deficits. This is particularly important if there is some level of cognitive impairment. History questions may need to be asked of a caregiver or family member if the older adult has little awareness of visual deficits. Table 8.1 provides a listing of pertinent vision history questions.

Several instruments have been developed to screen older adults for vision impairment. The Visual Function Index (Steinberg et al., 1994) is one instru-ment that has been used with community-dwelling adults to assess for visual impairment due to cataracts. Another visual function assessment instrument is the Activities of Daily Vision Scale (Mangione et al., 1992). Unfortunately, these instruments are helpful in specific disease states or settings and are not necessarily appropriate to all older adults, particularly those in long-term care. If a screening questionnaire is used, it should be determined if the instrument is appropriate for the setting and population of older adults being assessed.

Assessment of Visual Acuity

Visual acuity is the most commonly used measure of vision and is universally accepted as the method of measuring vision changes over time. Visual acuity is defined as the measurement of the ability of the eye to perceive the shape

TABLE 8.1 Visual Function History Questions

Are you experiencing any change in your vision?
When was the last time you saw your eye doctor?
How is your eyesight?
Do you know what your visual acuity was at your last eye doctor's
    appointment?
Are you experiencing any blurring in your vision?
Are you having any double vision?
Does light bother your eyes?
Does glare bother your eyes?
Are you having any eye pain?
Do you use any eye drops for dry eyes?
Do you use any eye drops for anything else?
Have you had any trauma or injury to your eyes?
Have you ever had any surgery on your eyes?
Do you have a family history of eye problems?
What changes have you made in your activities due to your vision?
If vision has changed, how has it affected your daily functioning?

of objects in the direct line of vision and to distinguish detail. Generally, it is tested by finding the smallest symbol on an eye chart that can be recognized at a given distance (Prevent Blindness America [PBA] & National Eye Institute [NEI], 2002). With aging, an individual has greater difficulty with visual accommodation, when the target of vision moves from near to far. This requires both the assessment of distance acuity and near vision acuity (Morse & Rosenthal, 1997). Visual impairment based on visual acuity has many definitions and varies widely around the world. The most commonly accepted definition of visual impairment is vision between 20/40 and 20/200, with vision less than or equal to 20/200 defined as legal blindness (PBA & NEI, 2002; Tielsch, Javitt, Coleman, Katz, & Summer, 1995).

There are several methods to assess distance vision in the older adult. Visual acuity is assessed most frequently using the Snellen chart or the Early Treatment of Diabetic Retinopathy Study Eye Chart (ETDRS), also known as the National Eye Institute, Ferris-Bailey Chart (Ferris, Kassoff, Bresnick, & Bailey, 1982). These tools measure distance acuity at the standard acuity levels of 20/10, 20/20, 20/25, 20/40, 20/80, 20/100, 20/200, 20/400, and 20/800. If the older adult is able to read the 20/30 line on the chart, but not the 20/40 line, vision should be retested using the pinhole test. The individual is asked to read the chart looking through a pinhole in a piece of cardboard. If vision is improved with this technique, it is quite likely a change in corrective lenses would improve visual acuity (Morse & Rosenthal, 1997; Schmidt Luggen, 2004).

There are many tools that measure near visual acuity. The Rosenbaum Near Vision Screener (Horton & Jones, 1997) is one of the most widely used measures. Another vision screener frequently used is the Lighthouse for the Blind Near Vision Screener, which has a 15-inch cord that allows for proper positioning of the visual screener (Lighthouse International, New York). One key element of achieving accurate visual acuity measurement is having adequate nonglare lighting. Illumination is the single most important factor in enhancing visual functioning (Wilkinson, 2003). Optimal illumination identified in a low-vision clinic was 1188 LUX, whereas normal home conditions had a median value of only 177 LUX (Silver, Gould, Irvine, & Cullinan, 1978). A LUX is the metric level of illumination measured on a work plane in a lighted space. Level of illumination is also described by foot candles (fc) and is measured with a light meter (Lightsearch.com, 2000). Visual acuity was improved in 82% of subjects by augmenting lighting in their home by adding a 60-watt bulb in a small adjustable lamp (Cullinan, Silver, Gould, & Irvine, 1979).

Visual acuity is affected by all major eye conditions associated with aging: presbyopia, cataracts, glaucoma, macular degeneration, and diabetic or hypertensive retinopathy. Distance acuity is essential for tasks, such as driving, scanning for safety hazards when walking, and participating in recreational activities. Assessment with the Snellen Chart, Early Detection of Diabetic Retinopathy Study Chart (EDDRS), or the Tumbling E chart will help determine an older adult's ability to navigate in the home environment by identifying problems with distance acuity.

Near visual acuity is essential for reading the written word, participating in hobbies and close work, as well as reading medication bottles. Assessment of near vision using an instrument, such as the Lighthouse Near Visual Acuity Screen (Elam, 1997; Lighthouse International) or the Rosenbaum Pocket Vision Screener (Horton & Jones, 1997), is important in the assessment of functional ability in the older person. Near vision is assessed in a well-lit environment holding the near vision acuity instrument 15 inches from the eye.

Assessment of Contrast Sensitivity

Visual acuity is measured under the best possible contrast levels using black contrasting print on a white background (Waiss & Cohen, 1991). The ability to distinguish beige from white is an example of a contrast that is not as marked, and greater contrast sensitivity is needed to differentiate these two colors. Contrast sensitivity measures the resolving power of the eye to discriminate an object from the background (Morse & Rosenthal, 1997). Most eye disorders associated with aging can impact contrast sensitivity, in addition to visual acuity.

Contrast sensitivity is not always included in a basic eye examination in ambulatory care or long-term care settings. However, adequate contrast sensitivity is very important in using appliances, turning on light switches, or identifying changes in a walking surface. Contrast sensitivity is also very important in distinguishing one pill from another when there are very subtle differences in contrast.

Assessment of contrast sensitivity can be completed using the Pelli Robson Contrast Sensitivity Chart (Pelli, Robson, & Wilkins, 1988) or the Vistech Contrast Sensitivity Test (Kennedy & Dunlap, 1990). These charts present letters or designs with progressively lower levels of contrast. Contrast sensitivity can be tested at 1 and 3 meters. These charts are subjective measures of a person's ability to detect low-contrast stimuli (Pelli, Robson, & Wilkins). Clinically, older adults often describe the designs or letters as faded.

Assessment of Fields of Vision

Fields of vision are described as the full extent of the area visible to an eye that is fixating straight ahead (Cassin, 2001). Adequate vision in all fields is important for safe navigation in the environment. Deficits in fields of vision can occur with cerebral vascular accidents (usually unilateral), glaucoma (peripheral fields), macular degeneration (central fields), or acute injury.

A gross measure of fields of vision can be assessed by the visual fields by confrontation test. This test is performed by the nurse, who sits facing the older adult at the same level about 18 inches apart. The older adult should cover one eye, and the examiner covers the opposite eye. The nurse extends his or her arm slowly, bringing his or her moving fingers from the periphery toward the center between the nurse and the older adult in all the six fields of vision. The nurse asks the older adult to report when he or she can see the nurse's fingers. The nurse then compares the older adult's ability to detect the fingers to his or her own ability, thus comparing the nurse's visual field with the older adult's. This exam requires the nurse to have intact visual fields. A more in-depth assessment, when deficits are identified, can be done in the ophthalmologist's office using a Goldman-type perimeter, a kinetic form of visual field testing, or by Humphrey Visual Field testing, which is a static type of perimetry (Gianutsos & Suchoff, 1997). Each of these techniques provides precise measurements of functional visual fields.

NURSING MODELS OF CARE FOR THE VISUALLY IMPAIRED

Nagi Disablement Process Model

Once deficits are identified in an older adult, nursing care must focus on determining how these deficits may impact functioning leading to disability. In

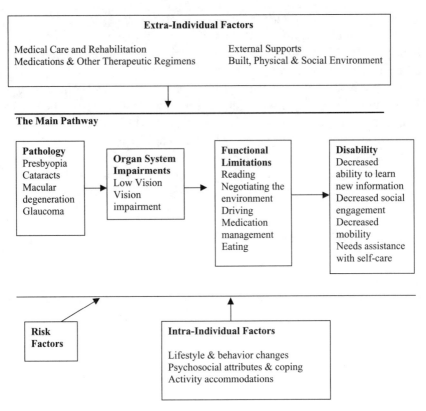

FIGURE 8.1 Nagi Disablement Process Model as adapted by Verbrugge and Jette (1994) applied to low vision.
Source: Reprinted from *Social Science Medicine, 38*, Verbrugge, L. M. & Jette, A. M. (1994). The Disablement Process, pp. 1–14, copyright 1994, with permission from Elsevier.

vision care, the goal is to prevent progressive visual impairment and blindness, and promote the use of adaptive techniques in those with chronic visual impairment and blindness that improve the quality of life. A method of conceptualizing how vision impacts older adults and causes disability is the Nagi Disablement Process Model (Nagi, 1991). Nagi describes the process of disability, which refers to the impact chronic and acute conditions have on the functioning of specific body systems and on an individual's ability to act in necessary, usual, expected, and personally desirable ways. The model has been adapted for application to those with vision loss by Verbrugge and Jette (1994) (Figure 8.1).

There are three major components that affect disability and outcomes according to the Nagi Disablement Process Model along a directional pathway: (a) the pathology that underlies the disease, (b) the level of organ system impairment induced by the pathology, and (c) the degree of limitation in functioning experienced by the individual resulting from pathological changes and organ system impairments. *Pathologies* may be defined as conditions such as presbyopia, macular degeneration, glaucoma, or cataracts. *Impairments* are specific structural abnormalities or conditions in a specific body system, such as decreased visual acuity, decreased contrast sensitivity, or a visual field deficit. *Functional limitations* refer to restrictions in performing fundamental physical and mental actions such as physical functioning and altered communication. *Disability* is a negative outcome and refers to reading difficulties, decreased cognitive performance, driving difficulties, and assistance required with dressing. This trajectory may have dire consequences such as acute confusion, falls, depression, and decreased quality of life for older adults with vision loss. Verbrugge and Jette (1994) describe extra-individual and intra-individual factors that can influence the pathway to disability.

The *extra-individual factors* can positively impact the pathway to disability. Nursing care to decrease disability outcomes includes assessment, nursing actions, and referrals for management of vision impairment. Medical care, such as cataract and laser surgery, and rehabilitation such as physical, occupational, speech and audiology therapy can decrease disability. Medications and therapeutic regimens, such as eye medications or antioxidants that may slow the progression of age-related macular degeneration, also can affect visual functioning. External supports such as nursing assistance and activity assistance will also assist the individual to maintain functioning and social interaction. The physical and social environment can play a large role in disability outcomes. Improving lighting, adding contrast to fixtures in the home, and improving access to care through better transportation may achieve improvement in the physical and social environment.

Risk factors include the predisposing characteristics of the individual that may lead to visual impairment. These would include such things as having a family history of glaucoma, blue eyes for macular degeneration, or having diabetes or hypertension. In older adults it is important to focus on pathological risk factors. *Intra-individual factors* include lifestyle and behavior changes, psychosocial attributes and coping, and activity accommodations. Examples of intra-individual factors are the type of coping mechanisms or personality type an individual has had all his or her life. These factors are considered to be the psychosocial aspects that the individual brings to the situation that can help or hinder functional ability.

The Sensory Enhancement Model

The Sensory Enhancement Model (SEM) is designed to guide nursing care to intervene on the negative trajectory identified by the Nagi Disablement Model. The Sensory Enhancement Model is a nursing intervention model that directs nursing care to the extra-individual factors from the Verbrugge and Jette (1994) adaptation of the Nagi Disablement Model. The Sensory Enhancement Model targets the extra-individual factors that impact uncorrected or uncompensated sensory impairment. The focus of the SEM is on the following extra-individual interventions: nursing assessment, nursing actions, and nursing referrals for medical care and rehabilitation (i.e., referral for cataract surgery, recreational therapy, and low vision center care), medications and therapeutic regimens, external supports such as adaptive equipment and devices, environmental changes such as improving lighting in the room, and social adaptations such as changing seating arrangements for dining and activities. These extra-individual interventions have been combined into a set of nursing interventions, the Individualized-Sensory Enhancement for the Elderly (I-SEE).

Individualized Sensory Enhancement for the Elderly

Nursing care for visually impaired older adults must be tailored to their type and level of sensory impairment. The I-SEE program provides a framework to guide nursing care. There are three steps of the I-SEE program: nursing assessment, nursing activities, and nursing referrals.

Nursing assessment is essential to individualizing the care of the visually impaired older adult. Asking the individual to describe any difficulty they may have with their vision may be helpful. Unfortunately, older adults may underreport their level of visual impairment. There are easy bedside screening techniques, such as near vision screeners and the pan ophthalmoscope that provide useful information related to impaired vision.

Nursing actions should be determined based on assessment of vision deficits. Examples of basic nursing actions in the care of older adults with vision impairment include:

- using voice or touch to get attention
- facing the older adult
- providing adequate lighting in the room
- routinely cleaning eyeglasses and other adaptive equipment
- removing clutter from the room
- providing lighted magnification
- enlarging reading materials using a copier
- using a large black marker for written instructions
- avoiding visual noise or visual clutter in the environment, such as numerous prints or pictures on the walls
- providing written instructions in at least a 14- to 16-point font on nonglossy, high-contrast paper
- reviewing medications for visual side effects
- administering prescribed eye drops

TABLE 8.2 Eye Drop Administration

- Wash and dry your hands. Put on clean gloves.
- Recheck eye drops to be sure you have the correct medicine, correct patient, and correct dose.
- Have the older adult lean back or look at the ceiling.
- Gently press below the lower eyelid along the bony prominence of the orbit of the eye to pull down the lower eyelid.
- With your other hand holding the eye medicine bottle with cap removed, gently squeeze the bottle to place one eye drop inside the lower lid. Administer the number of eye drops prescribed in each eye.
- After administration, apply pressure over the inner canthus against the bone for several seconds to occlude the puncta and minimize systemic absorption
- Gently dab away any excess medicine or eye drop fluid with a clean tissue.
- If two or more different eye medicines are required, wait 5 minutes between administrations.
- If the older adult has some cognitive impairment and will not participate in this method, administer the eye drops when the client is in bed lying on back. Provide warning that you are going to administer eye drops.
- Do not touch the eye medicine bottle tip to the eye.
- Recap the eye medicine bottle.
- Remove gloves and rewash and dry hands.

Source: Adapted from Web MD Medical Reference and The Cleveland Clinic. (2004). *How to insert eye drops.* Retrieved August 19, 2005, from http://my.webmd.com/content/article/63/71998.htm.

In a long-term care facility, eyeglasses should be kept clean and engraved with the older adult's name to avoid loss. Instilling eye drops for long-term care residents can often be complicated when a confused older adult is not able to be fully cooperative. See Table 8.2 for instructions on the correct instillation of eye drops. Successful nursing actions that facilitate care should be communicated within the visually impaired older adult's care plan.

Nursing referrals or requests for referrals to other disciplines can be important when caring for visually impaired older adults. Referrals to optometry or ophthalmology should be requested from the primary care provider for anyone who has not had their eyes examined in the last year, or if there is a reported acute change in vision or the presence of eye pain. Referrals to rehabilitation specialists (occupational therapist, physical therapist, audiologist, or low-vision specialist) should be made to assist older adults to use new assistive devices or to adapt to persistent vision impairment. Referrals to social services to assist with identifying community resources can also be helpful.

It is important to encourage older adults who are visually impaired to have communication partners to practice new skills and the use of adaptive equipment. The role of the communication partner is to facilitate the older adult's successful adoption of new sensory techniques through practicing the use of developing the proper environment for good visual contact (Tolson &

Stephens, 1997). Communication partners can be family members, nurses, or fellow older adults.

I-SEE takes into account the level and type of visual impairment when tailoring nursing interventions. If the interventions from the I-SEE are not sufficient to bring about positive change, expert assistance should be sought. The importance of attending to an older adult's visual status cannot be overstated. Many causes of visual impairment can be corrected, the progression slowed, and adaptations made. Nurses who ignore visual impairment, or accept it as normal aging, can contribute to a diminished quality of life for older adults with visual problems.

NURSING CARE OF EYE EMERGENCIES

Eye emergencies fortunately are not common, but they do occur in older adults. It is important to recognize their signs and symptoms and to refer for care immediately to preserve as much vision as possible. An older adult may not recognize vision changes as urgent, so a careful vision history is very important.

Retinal Detachment

A detached retina occurs when the sensory layer of the retina separates from the pigmented layer and may occur as a result of aging, hemorrhage, or trauma. Fluid seeps between the layers causing the retina to detach. A detached retina typically presents with a sudden or gradual increase in the number of floaters, flashes of light in the eye, or complaints of a curtain coming down in front of the eye (National Eye Institute, 2005). The prognosis for retinal detachments is good due to advances in laser surgery, if proper care is received. Older adults with these symptoms should see an ophthalmologist immediately, and if one is not available, they should go to the emergency room for treatment.

Acute Angle-Closure Glaucoma

Acute angle-closure glaucoma is fortunately not as common as open-angle glaucoma. Angle-closure glaucoma is secondary to the blockage of aqueous humor from flowing through the pupil into the anterior chamber of the eye. This increases the intraocular pressure behind the iris occluding the anterior angle chamber (Lee & Higginbotham, 2005). Acute angle-closure glaucoma is more common in people of Asian, Eskimo, or African American descent and presents with severe unilateral eye pain, blurred vision, colored halos around lights, and red eye. Headache, nausea, and vomiting can accompany vision loss (Plank, 2004). Older adults with these symptoms should be immediately referred to an ophthalmologist or the nearest emergency room to preserve their sight.

Temporal Arteritis

Temporal arteritis, also known as giant cell arteritis, is a granulomatous inflammation of the aorta and the aorta's proximal branches such as the cranial nerves. The inflammation of the temporal artery decreases the blood supply to the optic nerve. Temporal arteritis can cause sudden vision loss. Older adults with temporal arteritis may complain of scalp tenderness and headaches and may have jaw claudication causing pain with chewing, before the acute vision loss (Wooley, 2002). Those who describe these symptoms need to be evaluated by an ophthalmologist on an urgent basis, unless sudden vision loss accompanies the symptoms; then immediate evaluation is required. A better prognosis may be possible with immediate evaluation and treatment.

Cataract Surgery Complications

Cataract surgery has become very common in older adults. Complications are rare, but possible. Endophthalmitis following cataract surgery is a devastating infection of the anterior and posterior segment of the eye that may lead to blindness. Fortunately this complication is rare. The first week postoperatively is critical for monitoring for complications. The typical scheduled postoperative cataract surgery follow-up visit schedule is the day after surgery, 1 week after surgery, and again in 3 to 4 weeks (University of Washington Department of Ophthalmology, 2004). Nurses should monitor for complaints of increased pain or pressure in the eye, decreased vision, increased redness of the eye, or any drainage following surgery (Oetting, 2003). If these signs or symptoms occur, the older adult should return to their cataract surgeon immediately.

NURSING CARE BY SETTING

Home Care

Nursing assessment in the home setting provides insight into the older adult's functioning within his or her own environment for the purpose of developing individualized plans of care. Nurses can encourage those who are visually impaired to improve lighting in the home setting. Areas that should be addressed by the nurse in home care include adequate lighting, contrast in the home environment, and developing safe medication administration systems. Light bulbs should be at least 60 watts to provide adequate lighting for those with visual impairment. Contrast can be added to appliances, light switches, and changes in elevation, such as stairs, to provide safe mobility in the environment. Occupational therapy and physical therapy referrals, as well as referrals to low-vision clinics, may help facilitate the use of adaptive equipment appropriate for the functional level of those older adults who are functionally impaired.

Outpatient Clinic

Clinic nurses must be sure that the annual history and physical of each older adult includes adequate vision testing. Health promotion activities should include the monitoring of the older adult's visits to an optometrist or ophthalmologist. Educational materials for those with vision impairment should be presented on nonglossy paper with 14- to 16-font, high-contrast print. The clinic setting should also be free of safety hazards for visually impaired elders.

Acute Care

Acute care settings are potentially risky settings for older adults with vision loss because of the increased possibility of developing delirium (Inouye et al., 1999). When an older adult is ill enough to be in the acute care setting and is also limited by decreased visual function, there is a higher risk of confusion that may be decreased with the use of adaptive equipment, such as eyeglasses and lighted magnifiers that may allow fuller participation in self-care. Providing adequate lighting, large-font, high-contrast teaching materials, and mobility assistance as needed are a few areas that nurses can address in the acute care setting. Also in the acute care setting, the older adult and his or her family should be asked about routine eye medications. These are frequently omitted from the medication list on admission, but should not be missed.

Long-Term Care

The average age of long-term care (LTC) residents is estimated to be age 82.6, and over half of the elderly nursing home residents are 85 years of age or older (Sahyoun, Pratt, Lentmer, Dey, & Robinson, 2001). This older population is at great risk for chronic health problems such as glaucoma, macular degeneration, diabetes, and hypertension. In one study, over 50% of LTC residents were visually impaired at the 20/70 acuity level (Cacchione, Culp, Dyck, & Laing,

2003). Nurses in LTC must be cognizant that visual impairment is a significant barrier to the older adult's ability to fully engage in life in the LTC setting. It has also been estimated that as many as 54% of LTC residents have dementia (Magaziner et al., 2000), further compromising their ability to function independently. Eyeglasses and other adaptive equipment should be engraved with the resident's name and washed daily during morning care. Regular eye exams are recommended in LTC and all health care settings.

CARE PLANNING FOR THE VISUALLY IMPAIRED OLDER ADULT

As nurses provide care to older adults, nursing diagnoses are formulated which is a nursing judgment about individual, family, or community responses to actual or potential health problems/life processes. These nursing diagnoses provide the basis for selection of nursing interventions to achieve outcomes for which the nurse is accountable (North American Nursing Diagnosis Association [NANDA], 1999). Nursing interventions are behaviors, or nursing actions, that nurses perform to assist the patient to move toward a desired outcome. The success or failure of a nursing intervention is the nursing outcome. The linking of nursing diagnoses with nursing interventions and outcomes can serve as a useful model for planning care for low-vision older adults, as in the following case study.

CASE STUDY

Meet Ms. V.

Ms. V. is an 82-year-old female who was living at home with the support of a home health aide 4 hours daily. Ms. V.'s only daughter lives out of town but checks in frequently by telephone and visits for a weekend each month. The home care nurse came for her visit and noticed Ms. V. was having increasing difficulty walking in the home as she was bumping into objects on her right side. Ms. V. has mild cognitive impairment, but reported to the nurse that she was having increased difficulty with vision in her right eye. On a good day wearing glasses Ms. V. has distance visual acuity of 20/50 in her right eye and 20/70 in her left. When the nurse asked about any other problems, Ms. V. reported headaches that have been increasing in frequency and pain on chewing that started a few days ago. The nurse, using the I-SEE framework, performed a quick vision assessment using the Lighthouse for the Blind

Near-Vision Screener and checked visual fields by confrontation. Ms. V. had 20/800 vision in the right eye with markedly decreased visual fields. The nurse recognized this was an acute change in her vision and notified Ms. V.'s daughter. She also made a prompt referral to Ms. V.'s primary care provider, who sent her to the emergency room.

Ms. V. was diagnosed with temporal arteritis in the emergency room and immediately started on oral high-dose steroids and admitted for a temporal artery biopsy. When the daughter arrived at the hospital from out of town, she found her mother more confused than usual. The nurse in the hospital used the I-SEE framework to plan the care for this patient using the North American Nursing Diagnosis Association nursing diagnosis and the Nursing Outcome Criteria and Nursing Intervention Criteria. The nursing diagnosis was sensory/perceptual alterations: visual, and the first expected outcome of cognitive orientation required environmental management, safety surveillance, delirium management, communication enhancement, and cognitive stimulation. The second expected outcome was vision compensation behavior, which would require the use of adaptive equipment, environmental management, such as proper lighting and contrast, medication management for treatment of temporal arteritis, emotional support for the patient and her daughter, fall prevention, assistance with meals, and exercise therapy. The nursing interventions were identified using the I-SEE nursing assessment, actions, and referral framework. Ms. V. received daily vision assessment by the nursing staff. Nursing actions included providing adequate lighting in the room, removing clutter from the room, using voice or touch to get Ms. V.'s attention, using a large black marker for written instructions on high-contrast paper, and adding contrast to the fixtures in her room. Nursing referrals were made to a low-vision specialist and physical therapy.

Temporal arteritis was confirmed. Her vision improved significantly with steroid use. The nursing staff kept her safe and active during her hospital stay. Her confusion improved as her vision improved, and the steroid dose was maintained at 20 mg a day. She was able to return home within 3 days with increased nursing monitoring at home and a home health aide 4 hours a day.

Dual Sensory Impairment

Nurses are often confronted with difficulty communicating with older adults who have both vision impairment and hearing impairment. Older adults may compensate for the loss of one sense by relying more heavily on the other. If both vision and hearing are impaired, the older adult may become isolated, and the nurse's ability to care for the individual may be compromised. Hearing loss is very common and should be evaluated as one ages. The whisper test may be used as a screening assessment and is performed by having the older adult occlude one ear with a finger. In the opposite ear, the nurse, on a full exhale, whispers a three-syllable word such as ninety-nine. The older adult is then asked to repeat what the nurse whispered. This is repeated in the other ear. If the resident cannot hear the whispered voice, adaptations must be made, such as speaking in a lower voice and providing amplification.

Interdisciplinary Care

The nurse plays an important role in coordinating the interdisciplinary team and initiating referrals to appropriate disciplines. Referrals to an optometrist or ophthalmologist are important, but other referrals such as to occupational therapists, physical therapists, social services, and librarians may also improve the quality of life for older adults with vision loss. Occupational therapy is helpful in improving the individual's ability to perform activities of daily living, as well as recommending and training the individual on the use of special devices to make activities easier (Wilkinson, 2003). A physical therapist may be able to help with mobility and navigation issues associated with low vision, as well as self-protection training (Wilkinson). Social services help one to access professional and community resources, as well as provide support and assistance in coping with the social, functional, and emotional changes that may occur as a result of loss of vision, especially with the social changes that may occur due to the loss of vision (Wilkinson).

PREVENTING DISABILITY AND DIRE OUTCOMES OF LOW VISION IN OLDER ADULTS

Nursing care using the SEM and I-SEE can improve the quality of life of older adults with vision loss. Nursing assessments, actions, and referrals can greatly enhance the older adult's ability to effectively interact with his or her environment and the people around them. The I-SEE contains principles for identification of vision impairment, functional limitations occurring from the impairments, and preventing, when possible, the disability that may accompany the vision impairment. Even more importantly, individualized nursing care can help prevent the negative consequences that may result from vision impairment in older adults. By preventing disability from vision impairment and promoting quality of life through nursing assessment and individualized interventions, older adults can maintain functioning and prevent social isolation and other adverse outcomes that sometimes result in the older adult with vision loss.

REFERENCES

Cacchione, P. Z., Culp, K., Dyck, M. J., & Laing, J. (2003). Risk for acute confusion in sensory impaired, rural long-term elders. *Clinical Nursing Research, 12,* 340–355.

Cassin, B. (2001). *Dictionary of eye terminology.* Gainesville, FL: Triad Publishing. Retrieved June 24, 2005, from www.eyeglossary.net.

Cullinan, T. R., Silver, J. H., Gould, E. S., & Irvine, D. (1979). Visual disability and home lighting. *Lancet, 1*(8117), 642–644.

Elam, J. (1997). Analysis of methods for predicting near magnification power. *Journal of the American Optometric Association, 68*(1), 31–36.

Ferris, F. L., Kassoff, A., Bresnick, G. H., & Bailey, I. (1982). New visual acuity charts for clinical research. *American Journal of Ophthalmology, 94,* 91–96.

Gianutsos, R., & Suchoff, I. B. (1997). Visual fields after brain injury: Management issues for the occupational therapist. In M. Scheiman (Ed.), *Understanding and managing vision deficits. A guide for occupational therapists* (pp. 334–358). New Jersey: SLACK Incorporated.

Horton, J. C., & Jones, M. R. (1997). Warning on inaccurate Rosenbaum cards for testing near vision. *Survey of Ophthalmology, 42*(2), 169–174.

Inouye, S. K., Bogardus, S. T., Jr., Charpentier, P. A., Leo-Summers, L., Acampora, D., Holford, T. R., et al. (1999). A multicomponent intervention to prevent delirium in hospitalized older adults. *New England Journal of Medicine, 340,* 669–676.

Kennedy, R. S., & Dunlap, W. P. (1990). Assessment of the Vistech contrast sensitivity test for repeated-measures applications. *Optometry & Vision Science, 67*(4), 248–251.

Lee, D. A., & Higginbotham, E. J. (2005). Glaucoma and its treatment. *American Journal of Health-System Pharmacy, 62,* 691–699.

Lighthouse International, Low Vision Products, 36–02 Northern Boulevard, Long Island City, NY 11101.

Lightsearch.com (2000). Light guide: Lighting metrics: Quantity, quality, efficiency. Inter.Light, Inc. Retrieved August 1, 2005, from www.lightsearch.com/resources/lightguides/lightmetrics.html.

Magaziner, J., German, P., Zimmerman, S. I., Hebel, J. R., Burton, L., Gruber-Baldini, A. L., et al. (2000). The prevalence of dementia in a statewide sample of new nursing home admissions aged 65 and older: Diagnosis by expert panel. *Gerontologist, 40,* 663–672.

Mangione, C. M., Phillips, R. S., Seddon, J. M., Lawrence, M. G., Cook, E. F., Daily, R., & Goldman, L. (1992). Development of the Activities of Daily Vision Scale: A measure of functional vision status. *Medical Care, 30,* 1111–1126.

Morse, A. R., & Rosenthal, B. P. (1997). Vision and vision assessment. In J. A. Teresi, M. P. Lawton, D. Holms, & M. Ory (Eds.), *Measurement in elderly chronic care Populations* (pp. 45–60). New York: Springer.

Nagi, S. Z. (1991). Disability concepts revisited: Implications for prevention. In A. M. Pope & A. R. Tarlov (Eds.), *Disability in America: Toward a national agenda for*

Prevention (pp. 309–327). Division of Health Promotion and Disease Prevention, Institute of Medicine. Washington, DC: National Academy Press.

National Eye Institute. (2005). *Retinal detachment.* Retrieved August 29, 2005, from http://www.nei.nih.gov/health/retinaldetach/index.asp

National Institute of Health. (2002). *Healthy People 2010, Volume 2,* Vision and hearing. Retrieved August 1, 2005, from http://www.healthypeople.gov/document/HTML/Volume 2/28Vision.htm

North American Nursing Diagnosis Association (NANDA). (1999). *Nursing diagnoses: Definitions & classification. 1999–2000.* Philadelphia, PA: Author.

Oetting, T. A. (2003). Preventing and managing cataract complications: It takes a village. *Insight, 28*(1), 18–25.

Pelli, D. G., Robson, J. C., & Wilkins, A. J. (1988). The design of a new letter chart for measuring contrast sensitivity. *Clinical Vision Science, 2,* 187–193.

Plank, L. M. (2004). Head neck and face disorders. In L. Kennedy-Malone, K. R. Fletcher, & L. M. Plank (Eds.), *Management guidelines for nurse practitioners working with older adults* (2nd ed., pp.129–130). Philadelphia, PA: F.A. Davis.

Prevent Blindness America (PBA) & National Eye Institute (NEI). (2002). *Vision problems in the U.S.: Prevalence of adult vision impairment and age-related eye disease in America.* Retrieved August 18, 2005, from www.preventblindness.org/vpus/VPUS_report_web.pdf.

Sahyoun, N. R., Pratt, L. A., Lentmer, H. Dey, A., & Robinson, K. N. (2001). The changing profile of nursing home residents. 1985–1997. *Trends in Aging* (No. 2). Retrieved June 20, 2005, from www.cdc.gov/nchs/data/agingtrends/04nursing.pdf.

Schmidt Luggen, A. (2004). Sensory function. In P. Ebersole, P. Hess, & A. Schmidt Luggen (Eds.), *Toward healthy aging: Human needs and nursing response* (6th ed., pp. 347–377). St. Louis, MO: Mosby.

Silver, J. H., Gould, E. S., Irvine, D., & Cullinan T. R. (1978). Visual acuity at home and in eye clinics. *Trans Ophthalmological Society, 98,* 262–266.

Smeeth, L. (1998). Assessing the likely effectiveness of screening older people for impaired vision in primary care. *Family Practice, 15*(Suppl. 1), S24–S29.

Steinberg, E. P., Tielsch, J. M., Schein, O. D., Javitt, J. C., Sharkey, P., Cassard, S. D., et al. (1994). The VF-14. An Index of Functional Impairment in patients with cataract. *Archives of Ophthalmology, 112,* 630–638.

Tielsch, J. M., Javitt, J. C., Coleman, A., Katz, J., & Sommer, A. (1995). The prevalence of blindness and visual impairment among nursing home residents in Baltimore. *The New England Journal of Medicine, 332,* 1205–1209.

Tolson, D., & Stephens, D. (1997). Age-related hearing loss in the dependent elderly population: A model for nursing care. *British Journal of Clinical Practice, 49,* 243–245.

University of Washington Department of Ophthalmology. (2004). *Cataract surgery at the University of Washington.* Retrieved August 1, 2005, from www.depts.washington.edu/ophthweb/cataract.html

Verbrugge, L. M., & Jette, A. M. (1994). The disablement process. *Social Science Medicine, 38*(1), 1–14.

Waiss, B. W., & Cohen, J. M. (1991). Glare and contrast sensitivity for low vision practitioners. In R. London (Series ed.), *A structured approach to low vision care*: Vol. 3 (pp. 443–446). Philadelphia: Lippincott.

Web MD Medical Reference and The Cleveland Clinic. (2004). *How to insert eye drops*. Retrieved August 19, 2005, from http://my.webmd.com/content/article/63/71998.htm

Wilkinson, M. E. (2003). Low vision rehabilitation: A concise overview. *Insight, 28,* 111–119.

Wooley, D. C. (2002). Polymyalgia rheumatica. In R. J. Ham, P. D., Sloane, & G. A. Warshaw (Eds.), *Primary care geriatrics: A case based approach* (4th ed., pp. 643–648). St. Louis, MO: Mosby.

CHAPTER 9

Supporting Families of Older Adults With Age-Related Vision Loss

Catherine S. Sackett and Betsy Campochiaro

Nurses, more than most other people, recognize that when an older person has a chronic disease or condition, the impact of that problem extends far beyond the individual. The lives of family and friends are deeply affected for the long term with the consequences of chronic vision loss. The effective nurse extends care to the support system of the visually impaired adult and recognizes that nursing's scope of practice is ever expanding.

As the post-World War II generation ages into the retirement era, the sheer numbers of older adults who are at risk for age-related vision loss increases. Indeed, blindness and low vision may affect 1 in 28 persons over the age of 40 (The Eye Diseases Prevalence Research Group, 2004). Their care providers may include not only family but also friends and staff at assisted living facilities. With the increased mobility of modern society, close relatives who had traditionally provided care to older family members may not be readily available. Job transfers, retirement, and a host of other issues may separate the caregiver and the care recipient. The healthier aged often move to warmer climates for at least a portion of the year, leaving more than 70% of their frailer counterparts to live at home rather than in nursing care facilities (Watson, 2001).

The Inter-Parliamentary Union in Geneva made some very cogent points in its Resolution on the Health and Well-being of the Elderly in 1993. First among these was the recognition that aging is not synonymous with sickness and that old age and death are normal and natural stages of the life cycle. Among the many valuable ideas delineated in this resolution was the concept that aging is a lifelong process and that healthy lifestyles greatly enhance enjoyment of old age. Surely this has great relevance to older adults with impaired vision. Ideally as older adults enter the "golden years," they are able to look back over their lives and enjoy a feeling of accomplishment, to feel that their lives have been useful—that they have "made a difference." But for many older adults with low vision, their sudden loss of independence and productivity leads to depression and despair. They may enjoy good physical health but worry about becoming a burden to others.

HOW IMPAIRED VISION AFFECTS DAILY LIFE

Since 1900, life expectancy in the United States has increased dramatically. Today, the life expectancy at birth is 74.4 years for males and 79.8 for females in the United States (Arias & Smith, 2003). Longer survival rates mean otherwise healthy elders who suffer from any level of visual impairment have more at stake then ever before in preserving their vision. Nurses can play a pivotal role in assisting the families and friends of those with impaired vision to better quality and enjoyment of daily life.

The patient with vision impairment must be viewed within the context of his or her daily life. It is important to monitor the progression of vision loss and to determine whether the loss of vision is central or peripheral. Older adults may lose vision gradually, as with the slow constriction of a visual field. On the other hand, the deterioration can be shockingly rapid, as with a vitreous hemorrhage due to diabetic retinopathy or the development of a choroidal neovascular membrane in macular degeneration. Sometimes vision loss in one eye may not be discovered until the other eye is accidentally closed and the diminished vision is suddenly obvious.

Clues to the development of vision loss may also be detected by family members. A daughter may notice a sudden clash of colors in her mother's selection of garments. Dishes taken out of the cabinet may have bits of dried food clinging to them that have been overlooked by the older person with diminished vision. Bills may be overpaid or not paid at all because poor vision has confused the bill payer. A gradual loss of color sensitivity due to a slowly developing cataract may make distinguishing between navy blue and black difficult. Problems may present as relatively trivial annoyances, such as wearing a soiled blouse because the stain was overlooked. Important medical appointments may be missed because the person with impaired vision is no longer confident when driving and does not wish to bother family members with requests for rides.

Busy family members may be unaware of the depth and breadth of problems encountered by those who are vision impaired. There may be inability on the part of younger family members to relate to personal deficits of their older relatives. They may assume that Grandmother is just being difficult when she resists going to her granddaughter's wedding, unaware of the anxiety felt by this older woman in a social setting because of her loss of central vision. A woman with vision loss may be overwhelmed by the logistics of shopping for a new dress or getting her hair done. Worries about embarrassing herself or others by bumping into chairs in unfamiliar places or spilling food at the reception may be behind her decision to stay at home (Leinhaas & Hedstrom, 1994). She may feel totally alone in her visually limited world. It is difficult for others to comprehend the sense of isolation that older adults experience as a result of vision impairment. Health care providers may ask how the individual with vision loss is doing, and the automatic response may be positive despite the experience of frustration and isolation. Often, such an older person will feel intimidated and reluctant to describe his or her problems in the environment of a busy medical practice.

The older adult with vision loss who must earn a living outside the home has additional needs and concerns. Mistakes made in the workplace with the transposition of numbers or other discrepancies will be poorly tolerated by most employers. A truck driver whose vision is affected becomes disabled and may suffer not only financially but also may experience a loss of self-esteem as his ability to care for his family members is compromised. Of those people of working age with impaired vision, only 41.5% are gainfully employed (Leonard, 2002). Vocational rehabilitation will require tremendous courage on the part of the individual as well as consistent encouragement from family and friends.

Quality of life may be dramatically altered by impaired vision. Physical problems related to aging can worsen the impact of vision loss. Those older adults with hearing loss may have depended on an ability to lip read only to become more isolated when central vision is impaired. Limitations in mobility influence the ability to venture outside of the home and to interact with others socially and may increase isolation and loneliness. Vision impairment also increases the likelihood of falls and possible fractures. Often, those with low vision are only identified by therapists during rehabilitation after a fractured hip.

EMOTIONS AND VISION LOSS

Irreversible vision loss may be devastating to an older person as he or she realizes how the commonplace tasks performed in life are impacted. Regardless of the role, whether parent, grandparent, choir member, golfer, accountant, or photographer, every aspect of daily life may be affected by vision loss. Although intellectually a person may realize vision is impaired and there is no way to reverse the process, it does not necessarily mean that hope for improved sight is lost. The vision impaired eagerly await and sometimes pursue dramatic but unproven developments in both medicine and technology in the hope of vision restoration. Some patients with low vision will mistakenly believe that they have nothing to lose and will seek surgery that offers little promise of success. Researchers have found that hope and optimism are important (Moore & Miller, 2003). Even when an individual has accepted these limitations and is functioning well, there may still be periods when frustration mounts and anger is expressed. There will be days when even the best "adjusted" visually impaired person says "Why me?"

WHY SHOULD THE FAMILY BE PART OF THE TREATMENT TEAM?

Because vision impairment is usually permanent, the disability becomes a constant part of family life. How well the person with impaired vision is able to cope with impairment may be directly proportional to family involvement. Family lifestyle may change in many ways, some of them profound. Minor changes, such as furniture placement and lighting, may need altering so as to eliminate safety hazards. Major changes, such as relocation to a son or daughter's home or to an assisted living facility, may impact dramatically on family dynamics and finances. Family members may have to take time off from work to provide transportation to doctors' appointments. Research has shown that a positive approach by the family to the problems attendant to chronic disease provides better outcomes. A shared understanding of the multiple ramifications of compromised vision can result in a more positive outcome. As the family works together to provide support and addresses the issues related to vision loss, the older adult can gain autonomy and discover ways to function as independently as possible (Fisher & Weihs, 2000). If the patient perceives the family's response and interest as positive, he or she may be more open about personal needs and accepting help from family members.

HOW CAN THE FAMILY HELP?

The Scope of the Problem

The family needs to have a clear understanding about the cause of vision impairment, including severity and prognosis of the condition. The ophthalmologist, nurse, low-vision professional, and occupational therapist are important sources of information and assistance. A list of questions prepared ahead of the visit can be very helpful to family members. When the appointment is made, extra time should be requested by the family so that questions may be adequately addressed. A family member should accompany the older person to any appointment with a health care provider to provide support and ask questions the visually impaired older adult may not consider. Some older adults worry that if they use their eyes that they will "wear them out" and may walk around their homes with their eyes closed, "practicing being blind." Such misconceptions still persist and cause needless suffering. The scope of the disease process should be explained by the health care provider as well as its likely evolution. Some frequently asked and useful questions include, "How will my vision be affected? Is distance vision affected or only near vision? Is there distortion? Is color vision affected? What makes things better . . . or worse? Should I be able to see better on a cloudy day? Should my reading lamp be at shoulder level . . . below eye level?"

The intervention of family members during the interview with the ophthalmologist can be critical. Although the ophthalmologist may be unable to offer any therapies to improve vision, he or she is the chief referral source for rehabilitation and other support services. Although low-vision devices are still not covered, Medicare coverage for low-vision rehabilitation was approved in 2002 (Gieser, 2004). The family caregiver can use this opportunity to request referrals for vision rehabilitation counseling, support groups, and social services. Although the numbers of older adults with vision loss from age-related macular degeneration is high, referrals to vision rehabilitation lag far behind (Park, 1999). This underutilized service could help older persons with low vision maintain their independence.

There are informational videotapes available for older adults with low vision and their families. The National Eye Institute also has a number of publications available, which can provide valuable information about disease processes. This can be helpful as the older adult and his or her family plan for the future. Community agencies and hospital-affiliated groups may offer seminars and educational outreach programs.

Support groups can also offer valuable opportunities for both education and socialization. When family and patients are fully informed about the vision loss, they will be better prepared to function effectively, cope with changes related to low vision, and to anticipate caregiving problems.

Intervention Planning

The family and all members of the professional team (nurse, ophthalmologist, low-vision specialist, optometrist, and social worker) should take time to assess the needs and desires of the older person with a visual deficit, as well as those of the caregivers. A nurse may need to coordinate meetings between the professional team and the older adult and his or her family to reassess the plan of care. Reassessment of the plan should be performed regularly as the older adult and his or her family may have circumstances and needs that change.

Independence Needs

Often, older adults derive feelings of self-worth and well-being from functioning independently. The ability to maintain control over daily activities is very important to all, but especially to those with vision impairment. Sometimes relatively minor adjustments in daily habits can make a significant difference toward maintaining independence and promoting quality of life for the visually impaired. Creative approaches to daily chores may be as simple as having multiple strengths of magnifying glasses for different tasks. Sorting and storing clothing by color can help make garment choices easier. Denominations of money may be differentiated by placement in color-coded envelopes.

Socialization Needs

An older adult with vision impairment may experience social isolation with separation from his or her network of friends. This may result from the loss of driving ability or the relocation to the home of a son or daughter. Though surrounded by well-meaning family members, the older adult with vision loss may experience a sense of loneliness from the sudden absence of old friends and peers who have shared life experiences and memories. Researchers have reported that interpersonal relationships serve to promote a positive sense of self (Mitchell, 1990). Regular outings with friends, old and new, should be encouraged and arranged.

Finances

Tied closely to feelings of independence is the ability to manage one's own financial affairs. However, the older person with impaired vision may require someone to assist him or her in financial matters (Moore & Miller, 2003). Spouses or trusted family members are typically best suited for this role.

Creating a regular schedule to review mail and pay bills may alleviate some worries for an older adult with vision loss. The family member should ask how much of a payment the older person wishes to make on a credit card bill or if money should be set aside for vacations or holiday use. The person with low vision needs assistance in managing finances, not necessarily in decision making.

The use of a bold-tip pen and a check-writing guide may be very helpful for the older adult with impaired vision. Large print checks and bank statements are available. Adequate but glare-free lighting is a must. Some individuals with low vision may be very receptive to the use of the Internet for some banking and bill paying. There may also be software programs that will enable those with limited vision to function independently. Low-vision devices are available which can often be used successfully for financial record keeping. Income tax and property taxes may be lower for those with certain levels of vision impairment. These benefits should be explored. Adequate documentation of visual acuity status for tax purposes is important and may be obtained from the ophthalmologist.

Safety Issues

Adapting the home to provide a safer environment for those with vision impairment can be beneficial for the whole family. The old maxim "A place for everything and everything in its place" should be the guiding principle of re-organizing the family home. If the person with impaired vision can rely on consistent furniture arrangement, navigation of the home without accidental falling or tripping is more likely. Clutter should be kept to a minimum and walkways kept clear. The edges of steps should be marked with contrasting tape to prevent falls. General room lighting as well as reading lamps should be equipped with dimmer switches so that lighting may vary with the older adult's low-vision needs. Clear shower curtains may provide more light in the bathroom. Colored or floating soap may make bathing easier (Arends, 2003).

Cooking

There are several strategies that can be used in the kitchen to allow the older adult with low vision to cook. Placing spices and pantry supplies in a specific order will help him or her recreate favorite recipes with fewer mistakes. Marking frequently used temperature settings on the stove, oven, microwave, and other appliances with Velcro dots will allow reliable usage. Color-coded measuring spoons, tactile measuring cups, talking kitchen scales, combined with good lighting can make food preparation easier. Large-print cookbooks or recipe cards written with bold felt-tip pens will make reading recipes easier. Food served on contrasting colored plates (e.g., white rice on a green plate) may make mealtimes less stressful. Ice cubes, corks, or clean ping-pong balls can be used in a glass or cup to help the patient with visual impairment know when the glass is full. Measuring water before boiling rather than after can help to avoid burns.

Cleaning

Simplicity in house cleaning is best. Special possessions should be safely displayed or stored to forestall accidents. A lightweight upright vacuum cleaner or sweeper is less likely to trip an older adult than one with a long hose and wand. There are many multiuse environmentally friendly products that can be safely kept in the home. The use of caustic chemicals should be avoided. A feather duster can allow light dusting while decreasing the opportunities for breakage. Soft cotton gloves may be easier to use than a dusting cloth. A thoughtful and appreciated gift for the older adult with low vision may be a regular subscription to a cleaning service.

THE HEALTH OF THE FAMILY—THE PROCESS OF FAMILY EVALUATION

Although there are a number of resources available to the visually impaired and his or her family, this population remains underserved in terms of resources and support. Major tertiary care centers often have social work and rehabilitation departments to which referrals can be made. However, because many individuals with vision loss are treated for their eye disease and followed within the community, referrals may be delayed or never made, simply because the resources that would be in place in a large medical center are absent in a small ophthalmologist's office. Significantly the caregivers themselves, although vital participants in the daily care of the older adult with impaired vision, may have needs that could be easily addressed by the primary health provider but are often overlooked.

Identifying the Caregiver

In many families, when there is a chronic illness most of the care and planning will be provided by a single family member. The role of caregiver is not generally planned for in the same way as a career (Pearlin & Aneshensel, 1994). The need for caregiving may come suddenly or the role may evolve gradually. Generally the initial person to assume caregiving responsibilities will be the spouse. Daughters often assume the role when the aging parent is unable, for one reason or another, to continue.

When the initial diagnosis of an ophthalmic disorder is made and vision loss is at the earliest stages of development, the demands on the family members as caregivers may be minimal. The needs of the older adult may so gradually evolve that those caregivers closest to him or her may not notice that leisure time is being gradually occupied by caring for the older adult with low vision. For example, the formerly avid golfer may not realize that he hasn't played golf in 2 years because he didn't want his wife to feel left out of his plans. Guilt and resentment may gradually affect the well-being of the caregiver. It is not uncommon for caregivers to avoid reaching out to other family members when they need help. Some adults with low vision and their caregivers do not want to be perceived as "not coping" or needing help. Spouses may feel that the older adult with vision impairment and other disabilities or illnesses will perceive his or her condition as a weakness and will attempt to shield him or her from feeling embarrassed because of these functional impairments (McKeown, Porter-Armstrong, & Baxter, 2004).

Siblings may lash out in anger when there are no spontaneous offers of help from family members, who may retort, "It didn't look like you needed help!" As a result, the quality of life for the caregiver may also suffer. Shared burdens and problem solving help to ease the strain on the primary caregiver and can result in improved quality of life for the entire family.

Unfortunately, there is often no intervention until the family relationship deteriorates and a crisis ensues. The nurse may be the first person to ask the critical questions of both the person with low vision and the primary caregiver. Questions that should be explored with both the older adult with impaired vision and the caregiver include specific questions about activities of daily living, for example: "Who provides transportation for medical and social visits?" or "How are activities such as bill paying or grocery shopping handled?" Sometimes family caregivers may find themselves overwhelmed and frustrated without being able to identify the various sources of unhappiness and depression.

The Invisible Caregivers: Children

When the older person with low vision resides in the home of a son or daughter, other members of the family, including children and teenagers, may assume some of the caregiving responsibilities. Because so many women work outside of the home, school-age children may come home after school and find themselves helping a grandparent with his bills or identifying medications. Some children and adolescents may provide socialization and entertainment for the older adults, whereas others may be involved in more personal care. Although involvement in the care of a disabled family member can be a positive experience, the developmental age of the child should be considered. The nurse can alert the primary caregiver to unanticipated pitfalls and help avoid placing youngsters into situations for which they are unprepared (Lackey & Gates, 2001).

EFFECTS OF CAREGIVING ON HEALTH AND WELL-BEING

Emotional Stress

The ramifications of being the primary family caregiver are many and varied. Sometimes the caregiver grieves for the older adult with vision loss, feeling the loss acutely and sharing the emotional burden. Statements such as "He loved to read." or "Photography was his life! It's so unfair." are examples of burdensome and emotionally exhausting thoughts by the caregiver. At times the care recipient may berate the caregiver, charging him or her with a lack of sensitivity and sympathy, saying, "You just don't know or care how I feel." The mixed emotions and lack of understanding by the care recipient may increase the caregiver's stress. This may be evidenced by increased irritability, insomnia, and memory problems for the caregiver. Forgetting appointments or misplacing car keys can be warning signs that stress is building in the family caregiver.

Anxiety

Visual deficits of the older adult may predispose him or her to accident or injury. A loss of depth perception makes stumbling and falls more likely. An individual whose vision is borderline and who shouldn't be driving may worry family members by continuing to drive to the grocery store, endangering not only him but also others. Constant worry places increased stress on the caregiver and predisposes him or her to increased psychiatric morbidity (Schulz & Beach, 1999).

Multiple Roles

The person with impaired vision who previously maintained his or her home and attendant daily chores may have difficulty managing responsibilities with progressive vision loss. As a result, the family caregiver may need to assist. Taking care of finances, decorating the house at holidays, cooking, and shopping for gifts may all become new and perhaps unwelcome chores of the family caregiver. As these new tasks are assumed by various family members, tensions may arise because of individual differences in the manner by which these tasks are done.

Role changes between an adult child caregiver and an aging parent with impaired vision may be very stressful for both parties. The wife who assumes the role of caregiver for the husband may mourn the loss of her previous levels of social participation with her husband as partner (Seltzer & Li, 2000). She may be called on to enter the workforce or to assume household responsibilities that previously were the sole domain of her husband. A male spouse who suddenly finds himself responsible for grocery shopping or laundry may feel awkward and find he is unable to please his wife. The health of the spouse may not be robust and the strain of caregiving may lead to increased risk for health problems. Schulz and Beach (1999) have shown that prolonged caregiving and emotional strain in an older person is an independent risk factor for mortality.

Depression

There may seem to be no end to the care provided to older adults with chronic conditions because of the long-term nature of the health problem. Age-related vision loss is a chronic health condition. Stress may inevitably arise in even the most loving caregiver because of drastic changes in his or her lifestyle. Often the primary caregiver sacrifices his or her own needs for the sake not only of the impaired person but also for the rest of the family. When sacrifice leads to chronic emotional and physical fatigue, tempers fray and other negative feelings may occur. Insomnia, weight gain or loss, a feeling of hopelessness, a loss of interest in hobbies or thoughts of suicide may be symptoms of depression.

How a person reacts to the stresses associated with long-term caregiving may be dependent on a number of factors, including but not limited to gender, age, general health status, levels of fatigue, outside employment, recreational habits, and family support. Women report a higher rate of depression than do men, possibly because men may perceive depression as a weakness. Women, on the other hand, may be less likely to hire outside help, trying to do everything themselves, believing that they should be able to take care of the family. Those who work outside the home and try to run their own household, as well as that of an aging parent, will simply not have enough hours in the day to do both and may lose critical hours of rest. Sleep deprivation contributes to depression (Family Caregiver Alliance, 2004).

WHAT HELPS FAMILY MEMBERS?

Positive Aspects of Caregiving

Caregivers need to tell "their story." The nurse, more than the physician, may be perceived as someone to whom the caregiver can communicate. People involved in caregiving of long duration often have no one to tell about their experiences, to reinforce that they are doing a good job, and who can suggest solutions to problems. An important aspect of caregiving that should be discussed by the nurse is related to the positive aspects of caring for others. Cohen, Colantonio, and Vernich (2002) questioned study participants about positive aspects of caregiving that they had experienced. Seventy-three percent could cite at least one positive aspect of caregiving. Companionship (22.5%) and fulfillment/reward (21.8%) were mentioned most often. Those who are unable to identify any positive aspects of caregiving may be those at highest risk for depression and other subsequent negative health consequences. This may alert the nurse to those caregivers at highest risk for stress and depression.

Support Groups

Caregiver support groups enable people to share their frustrations and concerns with others who may be experiencing similar feelings. The opportunity to receive support from others who share similar feelings may be invaluable to family caregivers. A discussion of common problems may reveal innovative solutions.

A support group should have educational and social components. Information about available resources for the visually impaired and older adults and family members should be available. Group leaders should provide information about community resources, talking books, occupational rehabilitation, adult day care centers, low-vision centers, low-vision aids, catalogs, and computer software for low vision.

The educational component of these support groups should include information on the aging process, communication, problem-solving, stress management, conflict management, and socialization problems of older adults with low vision. A very important part of any support group for family members and caregivers should include stress assessment and the teaching of relaxation techniques.

The social component of a support group is vital. It facilitates a myriad of emotions to be expressed, ranging from anger, frustration, and guilt to relief expressed with tears and laughter. As the participants listen to one another's caregiving journey, each may express support to each other and realize through sharing that he or she is not alone. Morale is generally improved through such support group participation (Kaasalainen, Craig, & Wells, 2000). A sense of affiliation or belonging among support group members has been found to be very beneficial (Hardy & Rifle, 1993).

SEEKING SUPPORT EFFECTIVELY

Informal Help

Because of the gradual progression of dependency that can occur with age-related vision loss, family caregivers may not be aware of the changes in their own lifestyle as the demands of caregiving increase. Changes may only be noted when the stress level of the caregiver is at a breaking point. There are a number of impediments to providing help and support to the primary caregiver. The visual loss may be so gradual that the level of dependency may increase without the conscious realization of either party. The person with low vision may resist help from anyone but the primary caregiver because he or she may not want to reveal the extent of the visual impairment to other family members or friends.

A frank discussion with the low-vision older adult may reveal that there are strategies that could increase his or her ability to function independently, which in turn would decrease the stress on the family caregiver. Consultation with low-vision experts and follow-up and consistent encouragement can often enable the visually impaired person to learn new habits and to more effectively help themselves. Brody et al. (2002) describe a randomized clinical trial during which participants with age-related macular degeneration participated in a 12-hour self-management program over 6 weeks. At the conclusion of the program, improved independent function and decreased emotional distress were reported. Those participants who initially reported increased depressive symptoms were found to be less depressed at the conclusion of the trial.

The caregiver may be reluctant to ask for help for a number of reasons. There may be a feeling that asking for help reveals a lack of competence. Sometimes family members are simply unaware of what kind of help is needed. A caregiver who can make specific requests and outline expected or desired outcomes to family members may be more likely to receive needed assistance. For example, simply saying someone needs help doing Christmas shopping may not be explicit enough. Help may be needed making a list, determining preferences, shopping at the stores, making the purchases, bringing them home, and wrapping and labeling the gifts. More than one session may be needed to complete these tasks. The specifics of each request for assistance should be articulated so help with the essentials can be obtained.

Accepting that other people have their own styles and methods of helping can be a big step toward relieving the care burden on the primary caregiver. Being flexible in accepting assistance can relieve stress. Creating a list of specific areas where help is needed may encourage some family members and friends to pick those activities best suited to their talents and time. Those who are unable to provide help themselves may be willing to provide monetary assistance that will enable the provider to hire help. For instance, an adult son living in another town may agree to pay for regular lawn maintenance in the summer or seasonal housecleaning. An unemployed daughter may be willing to drive her visually impaired parent to medical appointments, the hairdresser, or to run errands.

Socialization is as important for the caregiver as it is for the visually impaired adult. Invitations to dinner or golfing or other recreational opportunities, often declined because of emotional fatigue or guilt, should be reconsidered. Responsibilities in caring for the older adult can result in social isolation for the caregiver. Having the freedom to leave the house and enjoy leisure activities can help to rejuvenate the caregiver's mental outlook.

FORMAL HELP

Provider Support

An often-overlooked relationship is that which potentially may exist between the caregiver and the care recipient's health care provider. The caregiver may sometimes be considered the "hidden patient" in the therapeutic relationship that exists with the health care provider. Ideally, the caregiver should receive some support from the provider that enables the caregiver to decrease stress and prevent depression. However, Musil et al. (2003) found that over time the support from the provider, as perceived by the caregiver, decreased for reasons that were not clear. It may be that over time the therapeutic actions offered by the provider are less effective as the patient's condition progresses. As the care recipient's condition worsens, perhaps other members of the health care team, such as nurses and occupational therapists, assume larger roles in the care partnership with the caregiver.

Respite Care

Adult day services can be an invaluable source of socialization for the visually impaired, thereby helping to relieve the caregiver of care responsibilities. Increasingly extended care facilities are making respite care available for non-residents for as short a time period as a 24-hour stay, to an extended stay of several days to weeks. Caregivers taking advantage of these facilities could be freed for vacations or business trips without fear of leaving a visually impaired family member alone. Some services also provide transportation, meals, day trips, and rehabilitative services.

Occupational Therapy

An occupational therapist that visits the home can make an assessment of needs and recommendations that allow the visually impaired person to remain within the home, pursuing a normal life with a few adjustments in routine and environment. An evaluation at a low-vision center followed by a visit to the home by an occupational therapist can be invaluable. A home visit with the older adult by the occupational therapist can help eliminate safety hazards and identify problem areas such as poor lighting, which can be modified to improve safe functioning. Low-vision devices may be borrowed from the low-vision center to evaluate their usefulness in the home setting.

Transportation

Some older adults are in assisted living communities that may provide transportation for shopping, appointment, and recreational activities. Many communities have Councils of Aging that provide bus transportation door to door. Insurance or Medicare may cover all or part of these commuting costs. Communities may depend heavily on charitable organizations, such as the United Way, the Lions' Club, or local church groups, to provide transportation assistance for older adults.

SUMMARY

The goal of nurses who care for the older adult with impaired vision should be to minimize loss for individuals and their caregivers. Ongoing support of family caregivers is a critical role of the nurse. Nursing interventions that enhance the relationship between the visually impaired and the family caregiver will promote the quality of life for all and result in satisfaction for the nurse. By supporting families of older adults with low vision, the nurse is often the pivotal health care provider to whom the patient and his or her family may turn with confidence.

REFERENCES

Arends, C. (2003). *Good ideas for low vision patients*. Wheaton, IL: Edwin and Lois Deicke Center for Visual Rehabilitation.

Arias, E., & Smith, B. (2003). Deaths: Preliminary data for 2001. *National Vital Statistics Reports: From the Centers for Disease Control and Prevention, National Center for Health Statistics, National Vital Statistics System, 15*(5), 1–44.

Brody, B. L., Roch-Levecq, A.-C., Gamst, A. C., Maclean, K., Kaplan, R. M., & Brown, S. (2002). Self-management of age-related macular degeneration and quality of life: A randomized controlled trial. *Archives of Ophthalmology, 120*(11), 1477–1483.

Cohen, C. A., Colantonio, A., & Vernich, L. (2002). Positive aspects of caregiving: Round out the caregiver. *International Journal of Geriatric Psychiatry, 17*, 184–188.

The Eye Diseases Prevalence Research Group. (2004). Causes and prevalence of visual impairment among adults in the United States. *Archives of Ophthalmology, 122,* 477–485.

Family Caregiver Alliance. (2004). *Caregiving and depression.* Retrieved July 12, 2004, from http://www.caregiver.org/caregiver.

Fisher, L., & Weihs, K. (2000). Can addressing family relationships improve outcomes in chronic disease? Report of the National Working Group on Family-Based Interventions in Chronic Disease. *The Journal of Family Practice, 49,* 561–566.

Gieser, J. P. (2004). When treatment fails: Caring for patients with visual disability. *Archives of Ophthalmology, 122*(8), 1208–1209.

Hardy, V., & Rifle, K. (1993). Support for caregivers of dependent elderly. *Geriatric Nursing, 14,* 200–204.

Inter-Parliamentary Union. (1993). *The health and well-being of the elderly.* Resolution of the 90th Inter-Parlimentary Conference. Retrieved January 16, 2005, from http://www.ipu.org.

Kaasalainen, S., Craig, R. N., & Wells, D. (2000). Impact of the Caring for Aging Relatives Group Program: An evaluation. *Public Health Nursing, 17*(3), 169–177.

Lackey, N., & Gates, M. (2001). Adults' recollections of their experiences as young caregivers of family members with chronic physical illness. *Journal of Advanced Nursing, 34*(3), 320–328.

Leinhaas, M.-A. M., & Hedstrom, N. J. (1994). Low vision: How to assess and treat its emotional impact. *Geriatrics, 49*(5), 53–56.

Leonard, R. (2002). *Statistics on vision impairment: A resource manual.* New York: Arlene R. Gordon Research Institute of Lighthouse International, The Lighthouse Inc.

McKeown, L. P., Porter-Armstrong, A. P., & Baxter, G. D. (2004). Caregivers of people with multiple sclerosis: Experiences of support. *Multiple Sclerosis, 10,* 219–230.

Mitchell, G. L. (1990). The lived experience of taking life day-by-day in later life: Research guided by Parse's emergent method. *Nursing Science Quarterly, 3,* 29–36.

Moore, L. &, Miller, M. (2003). Older men's experiences of living with severe visual impairment. *Journal of Advanced Nursing, 43*(1), 10–18.

Musil, C. M., Morris, D. L., Warner, C. B., & Saeid, H. (2003). Issues in caregivers' stress and providers' support. *Research on Aging, 25*(5), 505–526.

Park, W. (1999). Vision rehabilitation for age-related macular degeneration. *International Ophthalmology Clinics, 39*(4), 143–162.

Pearlin, L. I., & Aneshensel, C. S. (1994). Caregiving: The unexpected career. *Social Justice Research, 7,* 373–390.

Schulz, R., & Beach, S. R. (1999). Caregiving as a risk factor for mortality: The Caregiver Health Effects Study. *The Journal of the American Medical Society. 282*(33), 2215–2219.

Seltzer, M. M., & Li, L. W. (2000). The dynamics of care giving: Transitions during a three year prospective study. *The Gerontologist, 40*(2), 165–178.

Watson, G. R. (2001). Low vision in the geriatric population: Rehabilitation and management. *Journal of the American Geriatrics Society, 49,* 317–330.

CHAPTER 10

Assistive Devices and Resources for Older Adults With Age-Related Vision Loss

Betsy Campochiaro and Catherine S. Sackett

Older adults with low vision often experience an accompanying sense of isolation and helplessness. Severe sight loss is a risk factor for a person's ability to carry out everyday activities. This can lead to a myriad of emotional responses, particularly depression (Hinds et al., 2003; Rovner & Casten, 2002). In one study, 33% of adults with bilateral macular degeneration had clinical depression, which is two times the rate of depression in older adults without macular degeneration (Gieser, 2004). Depression can hinder the ability of individuals to seek help from others, and it has also been associated with a decline in self-reported vision independent of actual change in visual acuity (Rovner, Casten, & Tasman, 2002). These are compelling reasons for nurse intervention at the time of diagnosis. The impact of education and support has been demonstrated to effectively increase independence and improve mood and function of the older adult with vision loss (Brody et al., 2002). The nurse is in a unique position to help individuals adjust to this condition by providing avenues to learn new ways to perform everyday activities that may assist in regaining their prior sense of well-being. Learning to live and function independently, despite having low vision, is the goal of rehabilitation. This can start with the nurse. The nurse can be the pivotal person, not only to provide the emotional support but also to introduce patients to organizations and numerous other resources that can help older adults with the burden of overcoming their disability.

LOW-VISION REHABILITATION

The health care provider should introduce vision rehabilitation early, as this is a critical component in the management of vision loss. Speedy referral to a low-vision center is one of the first steps in assisting patients to manage and adjust to low vision. Low-vision rehabilitation can help older adults with visual disabilities that suffer from a loss in functioning in activities of daily living. It can also be helpful to those whose anxiety and depression hinder the adjustment process (Greenblatt, 1989; Margrain, 2000; Schuchard, 1999).

The nurse managing patients with low vision should be familiar with and play a major role in the rehabilitation process, to ensure the older adult with vision loss receives the information and tools necessary to live full and independent lives despite their visual handicap (Scott, Smiddy, Schiffman, Feuer, & Pappas, 1999).

WHAT IS LOW VISION?

A person with low vision is anyone who has permanent partial sight due to eye diseases, strokes, or accidents that is not correctable with spectacles, lenses, or surgery (Scott et al., 1999). It is commonly accepted that those individuals whose visual acuity is 20/60 or less in the better eye have low vision. Severe visual field loss may be another indicator of low vision despite a visual acuity better than 20/60. Color contrast and night blindness are other deficits that can occur within the definition of low vision. There are an estimated 2.4 million people in the United States with low vision. The leading causes are age-related macular degeneration (54.4%), cataracts, and glaucoma (The Eye Diseases Prevalence Research Group, 2004). These numbers are expected to rise due to the increasing number of aging adults.

THE REFERRAL PROCESS

The first step in the rehabilitation process is timely referral to a rehabilitation team. The ophthalmologist is considered to be the gatekeeper of low-vision services (Greenblatt, 1989). Ideally the ophthalmologist will recognize the need for referral at the point low vision is inevitable. This can be before the clinical criteria for low vision are met in anticipation of the future needs of the older patient. For example, it may be much easier to learn keyboarding skills with good vision than with poor vision. If the vision prognosis is poor, it would be to the benefit of the patient to introduce the concept of vision rehabilitation and the availability of opportunities before low vision occurs. Although this may produce anxiety in the patient, a frank explanation of the prognosis may motivate the patient to gain skills in preparation for potential vision loss. In a study done by The Lighthouse, only 43% of those individuals surveyed who were affected by vision loss, either themselves or a family member, knew of low-vision services in their community (Scott et al., 1999). People are unaware of these services due in part to the lack of referral.

The National Eye Institute (NEI) launched a program in October 1999 to address the lack of education and assistance individuals need to successfully adjust to low vision. Recognizing the implications of low vision on individuals' lives, the NEI program emphasizes the importance of the rehabilitation program. It addresses the information gap that exists with individuals with low vision, the public health community, and the research community (Kupfer, 2000). Providing the patient with opportunity for assistance can improve adjustment to low vision. Vision rehabilitation can also assist those with less severe vision loss to deal with the frustration of completing everyday tasks or coping with the fear and anxiety of vision loss. Increasing competency and support will provide the older adult with the necessary skills for independent living.

Referral for low-vision services may not be made if the ophthalmologist focuses only on the medical management of disease and does not consider all the needs or spends little time listening to the patient. Although physicians may not spend the time necessary to manage nonmedical interventions for the older person with vision loss, nurses can and should educate the patient and family. It may be assumed that the nurse has more time than the physician to listen, so the older adult may be more comfortable describing to the nurse difficulties encountered related to vision loss. A few minutes of empathetic listening may reveal a myriad of problems that may go unstated if the elderly patient feels rushed. The nurse can also observe the patient with family members, which may provide clues about unmet needs. Given concerns about unmet needs, the nurse may become aware for the need to institute the referral process at any point in the care continuum.

Assessment for referral to low-vision services should always be made at the initial office visit, as well as at follow-up visits, to determine whether the older adult is psychologically ready and would benefit from vision rehabilitation services. A short series of questions can be asked of the patient to determine if referral would be helpful. These questions should address concerns about the present living situation. Are there family members or friends to assist with difficulties? What are the problems in functioning related to daily activities? How often does the older adult get out of the home? Who drives? Does the patient continue to travel? Does the patient pursue any special interests? Does the patient understand the vision loss? Does the family understand? Are there any signs of depression? Who is in the support network (Greenblatt, 1989)? Sensitivity to individuals that may not be forthcoming with information can help identify those who may benefit from rehabilitation services. If any responses from the aforementioned questions convey struggles or loss of function, the nurse should initiate the referral process.

During the evaluation period, realistic outcomes of the eye disorder should be discussed. For example, macular degeneration does not result in total vision loss. A return to full functioning may be possible with education and support. False hopes, such as complete reversal of vision loss, will only delay the acceptance of visual disability. Sensitive, open, and reassuring discussions may provide hope at a time of great anxiety and despair (Fletcher, 1994).

An important factor in the initial assessment for low-vision services is to determine whether the older adult meets the definition of legal blindness. If this definition is met, the older adult would be in a better position to benefit from a variety of comprehensive services and sources of financial assistance that are specifically for the blind and visually impaired. These services are more affordable due to a diagnostic status of legal blindness. Once the older adult meets the definition for legal blindness, it is imperative to carefully explain why this term is necessary and what it means for the management of services. The patient should understand that it is a qualifying definition used to register the patient for eligibility for state services. It does not mean the he or she will lose all sight and become completely blind (Greenblatt, 1989). Legal blindness is defined as central vision or acuity of not more than 20/200 in the better eye with all possible correction or a visual field constricted to 20 degrees diameter or 10 degrees radius.

THE REHABILITATION TEAM

Once the older adult with vision loss is in the rehabilitation system, there are a number of professionals on the team that can assist in the promotion of independence. A brief overview of the role of each team member is provided to help clarify the range and depth of services and resources offered by this valuable group of professionals.

- Nurse—provides assessment and referral, education, emotional support, case management, and home visits.
- Social worker—provides financial planning, emotional support, and referral management.

- Occupational therapist—provides home visits for safe functioning and ADL education.
- Rehabilitation counselor—coordinates services, develops plan of action, and sets attainable goals.
- Rehabilitation teacher—provides individualized instruction, skills development, and practical adaptations in the home and at work.
- Orientation and mobility instructor—develops safe travel techniques, instructs on use of the cane, and encourages increased awareness of surroundings through the use of remaining vision and other senses.
- Psychotherapist—aids in the emotional adjustment to low vision and addresses barriers to independence.
- Ophthalmologist—provides medical care and treatment and initiates the rehabilitation process. If employed in the low-vision center setting, may have expertise in prescribing optical and nonoptical devices.
- Optometrist—assesses visual function and recommends devices and appliances.
- Self-help groups—provide a forum for education, support, and emotional adjustment for the patient and the family.

Although all these professionals may not be represented at every low-vision center, a center of high quality will combine roles to provide the visually impaired older adult with all the necessary services he or she may need.

THE LOW-VISION ASSESSMENT AND PLAN

The low-vision assessment is the first step taken in the rehabilitation process. A lengthy interview is performed to determine the current level of functioning and to pinpoint the main problems the patient is experiencing in everyday living. This comprehensive review will also reveal any social or emotional difficulties that may not be initially evident. The interview is followed by a clinical exam and functional assessment. The clinical exam consists of distance/near acuities, retinoscopy, tonometry, slit-lamp biomicroscopy, visual field testing, color vision testing, contrast sensitivity, and evaluation of low vision. The functional assessment includes functional visual acuity and fields, color contrast discrimination, ocular motor skills, lighting, use of visual and nonvisual cues, and performance of activities of daily living (ADLs) (Watson, 2001). The evaluation and results of this assessment culminate in a vision rehabilitation plan. This plan summarizes the individualized rehabilitation goals and objectives. Recommendations are made by the low-vision team for devices that the adult with low vision may find helpful to assist in attaining the goals and objectives.

These recommendations may also include referral to other professionals such as a psychiatrist, occupational therapist, driving instructor, and/or support group. The rehabilitation process begins, and the adult with low vision meets regularly with the therapist until proficiency is attained with the recommended devices and the goals and objectives of the treatment plan are met.

Vision rehabilitation therapy has been documented to improve patients' ability to perform tasks, reading ability, and general level of independence (Gieser, 2004; Stelmack, 2001). This may improve overall life satisfaction and quality of life. Referral to a low-vision clinic is critical for the well-being of the older adult with vision loss.

AIDS AND TECHNIQUES

Sighted Guide

Any individual that assists an older adult with low vision should be familiar with the best method of leading a visually impaired person around unfamiliar territory. Nurses can easily teach this technique to family members and significant others. The individual assisting the individual with low vision is the sighted guide. This person should walk several steps ahead and have the person with low vision grasp his or her elbow. This technique allows the older adult with vision impairment to anticipate changes in levels by sensing the guide's up-and-down movement. The individual needing assistance should never be pushed or pulled when ambulating.

Canes and Guide Dogs

Although the majority of older adults with vision loss are not blind or without any usable vision, many could benefit from the use of a cane or a guide dog. Although there may be stigma associated with using these techniques, once the older adult is aware of the benefits and ease of use, the stigma can be overcome and safe navigation may be improved. The use of a white cane should indicate to others that vision is impaired. Because of this, others may offer assistance more readily. Assistance, however, may be used selectively in some circumstances. The use of the cane can greatly increase independent travel. Training is required and is provided at low-vision centers. The use of a guide dog can be an alternative to the cane for older adults with minimal remaining sight. A guide dog requires more responsibility and expense, not only in caring for the dog but also in training to work with a guide dog. The training usually occurs at guide dog schools, which are located throughout the country.

Optical Aids

Not all optical aids assist everyone in every situation, so the selection of an aid should be individualized for each older adult with vision loss. Different aids are appropriate for different types of activities. Although finding the right combination of devices for each individual is an important step in the rehabilitation process, educating the older adult to use the device(s) is challenging for the low-vision provider. Perseverance, patience, and flexibility are needed to incorporate new devices and techniques into everyday living. The nurse can assist the older adult with encouragement and support during follow-up visits. Some of the most common devices that are prescribed by a low-vision specialist may be organized under two main categories: magnification and lighting.

Magnification

The amount of magnification required is determined by one's visual acuity. There are different strengths of magnification for different uses. For example, magnifiers are available for close-up work and distance. Finding the best magnifier for a particular task requires experimentation with the different strengths. It may be beneficial to recommend having several types of magnifiers in the house to meet the demands of everyday living. There are several types of magnifiers that are important to consider:

- A portable hand magnifier is useful for spot reading, such as price tags and telephone numbers. It can hang from the neck or fold for easy storage. These magnifiers may be illuminated, which is particularly helpful for dark restaurants or anyplace where lighting is inconsistent.
- A stand magnifier is effective for continuous reading such as cookbooks, mail, and novels. This type is especially useful for older adults who have tremors or arthritis, making it difficult to hold the magnifier.
- A head-mounted magnifier is recommended for hands-free work, like knitting or sewing. These magnifiers may be lenses that are mounted on spectacles.
- A distance magnifier such as a telescope is useful for viewing street signs, house numbers, or airport gates.

Magnification can also be in the form of video magnification or closed-circuit televisions (CCTV). This is a stationary desk-type unit that has a screen monitor and a camera. Items placed under the camera are projected to the screen where the color, contrast, and image size may be manipulated for the best viewing for the individual. This device makes it possible for individuals with a visual acuity of less than 20/400 to read books, newspapers, and mail; and write checks and view photos. These devices are very expensive to purchase; a black and white unit may start at $1,800. This device should not be purchased without the assistance or advice of a low-vision specialist and only if it can be used for a trial period and returned if necessary.

Advances in technology and competition among manufacturers of low-vision equipment have resulted in a new product: a smaller, portable, closed-circuit video magnifier. This piece of electronic equipment provides variable magnification and contrast for reading and writing of printed material. The units allow the user to perform tasks outside the home, such as reading a menu or product labels. The units are powered by electric current and battery, which will last typically 2 hours before needing to be recharged. The viewing screen is part of the unit. Each device has variable features including level of magnification, field of view, weight, and color. The price can range from $900 to $2,500 depending on the unit and features (Deremerick, 2003).

Computer advances have facilitated the ease of computer use by older adults with low vision. Software is now available that can magnify the information on the computer screen. This magnification will cause there to be a smaller field to view on the screen. If this is bothersome, the software can enlarge just parts of the screen. It may be that only a section such as a toolbar may need magnification.

Some software programs can change the contrast to improve visibility of the fonts. For example, the lettering could be white on a black background or black lettering on a white background. Although these two options are most preferred by older adults with low vision, color contrast is also available, for example, green lettering on a black background. Due to individual preferences, it is best to try several combinations before deciding which option to use.

Other software comes bundled with the options for screen readers along with the magnification, thus making it possible for a voice to read the text and describe icons and photos. Another type of software called voice recognition allows the user to speak commands into the computer rather than keystroking. These innovations allow the older adult to have access to information on the Internet and communicate with e-mail. Training is required for most programs, but with a few good hours of investment, the majority of older adults will be able to master these programs. See the list of resources for suggested software.

Illumination

Reading ability is enhanced with better lighting for the older adult with low vision. As one ages, light demand increases by two to three times, and glare may become more problematic due to cataracts. The following list identifies several methods for the older adult with low vision to reduce glare and improve lighting.

- A small goose-neck-type lamp with an indoor floodlight bulb can be moved around the house, directing the flood of light where it is needed and away from the eyes to reduce glare.
- All the incandescent light bulbs in the house can be changed to 100 watts.
- A flashlight can be made readily available for extra light.
- Windows can be covered with sheer curtains to reduce sun glare in the home.
- All surfaces that are shiny and polished could be covered to reduce glare (i.e., floors with rugs and tabletops with cloths).
- NOIR glasses may be worn; these glasses have a yellow tint and can be worn alone or over prescription glasses to reduce glare.

NONOPTICAL AIDS

There is a wealth of nonoptical aids that include simple modifications with which the nurse should be familiar. The nurse should encourage the older adult with low vision to use nonoptical aids to maintain the highest level of functioning possible.

A bold pen with bold lined paper may improve visibility of written notes. Writing guides, which are plastic overlays, are available for check writing and signatures. Large-print checks can be ordered from banks, as well as large printed statements. There are talking clocks, watches, calculators, telephones, and scales. Kitchen gadgets talk as do TV remote controllers, and these tools can be especially helpful for the older adult with low vision. Patients may appreciate knowing about large-print books, cookbooks, and magazines.

The use of color contrast everywhere in the home should be encouraged. Dark switch plates for lights on a pale-colored wall, a dark chopping board for dicing vegetables, and solid dark-colored dishware on light-colored placemats are just a few examples of color contrast use in the home. These items are readily available from catalogs such as *Maxiaids* or *Independent Living Aids, Inc.*

Organizational strategies can be extremely helpful for the person with low vision. Having a place for everything provides familiarity, comfort, and security. Organizing clothing by color, labeling canned goods and medicines with nail polish, and using Velcro for frequently used buttons on stoves, microwaves, and washer and dryers will make vision loss less of a problem for everyday living. Safety issues should be addressed such as cabinets left partially opened and kitchen chairs left out of place. Attention to details can prevent falls and accidents.

THE NURSE'S ROLE IN EDUCATION AND SUPPORT

Although there has been substantial progress in the development of new treatments for many diseases contributing to low vision, for the majority of older adults with low vision, there are few medical or surgical interventions that will restore or prevent loss of vision. This does not mean that these older adults are beyond help. On the contrary, it is critical that nurses address the many problems created by vision loss, which is a major life-changing event. This devastating disease threatens the independence and well-being of older adults, filling their final years, which should be a time of reflection and fulfillment, with frustration and depression. The diagnosis of any disease that threatens vision is often accompanied by fear of total blindness, lack of understanding, feelings of helplessness, embarrassment, and a sense of isolation, all of which may negatively impact many aspects of the aging person's life. Although the medical community may not be able to restore or prevent vision loss through current therapies, the nurse is in a unique position to strengthen the individual's and family's ability to adjust to low vision. Nurses can effectively initiate the educational process through contact with the older adult and family, as well as referral to appropriate resources and organizations. This critical intervention may be the vehicle to acknowledge and address the needs of the older adult with vision loss. This educational and supportive approach enhances the well-being and competence of the patient with low vision and the family (Brody et al., 2002). The individual who has been diagnosed with a progressive and degenerative loss of vision such as macular degeneration often leaves the physician's office with many unanswered questions. The older adult may react with shock and disbelief, fearing the impact this diagnosis will have on his or her future. Questions regarding his or her specific condition may not occur to the older adult or family until after they are home. Nurses can provide the older adult and family with much-needed information in a more relaxed setting. This can occur in the everyday interactions with patients or within the context of a support group setting. Finding ways to normalize vision loss and incorporate it into a sense of well-being are important areas to address. The use of support groups specifically for adults with low vision provides time to get questions answered, meet others in the same condition, learn about disease processes, and improve ways of coping (Brody et al., 2002; Dahlin-Ivanoff, Klepp, & Sjostrand, 1998).

Increasing disease comprehension through structured patient/family education forums has been shown to increase the competence of older adults through active participation in the treatment and adjustment process (Davison, Pennebaker, & Dickerson, 2000). Improved knowledge about diseases can reduce delay in seeking help which, given the narrow time frame for targeted therapy for age-related macular degeneration, can be the crucial influencing factor for preventing vision loss. The patient and family's understanding of the disease process can improve communication about the needs and frustrations of all in the family. Family support was found to be a powerful predictor for continued use of low-vision devices in a study done with veterans diagnosed with macular degeneration (Watson, 2001).

The diagnosis of irreversible vision loss often forces major changes in family lifestyle, which may change the allocation of power, personal autonomy, role functioning, and decision making. The independent, outgoing husband may become depressed and unable to make the necessary adjustments to living with low vision. This puts more responsibility on caring family members to assist in daily living and to provide encouragement and optimism for living beyond the disease. Education can enable families to own diseases jointly rather than thinking of it as solely a problem of the patient. This sharing and understanding within the family has been shown to affect the physiologic functioning of the patient and the behavioral and emotional lives of all family members. This can positively affect outcomes in adjustment and management of disease (Davison et al., 2000).

The following reference list has been developed to facilitate the nurse in the role of educator. The method of education, whether the nurse chooses a formal, structured group or a more informal one-to-one interaction with the older adult, is not as important as the actual process of interchange. This exchange is vital to the adjustment to low vision. With the following resources, the nurse can initiate referral and follow-up, as appropriate, for the level of vision loss. This will provide the older adult with the tools necessary to lead an independent and fulfilling life.

RESOURCES

American Academy of Ophthalmology
P.O. Box 7424
San Francisco, CA 94120-7424
(415) 561-8500
http://www.eyenet.org
This organization provides brochures on low vision and other eye problems as
well as helps locate ophthalmologists throughout the country.

American Council of the Blind
1155 15th Street, N.W., Suite 720
Washington, DC 20005
(800) 424-8666
(202) 467-5081
http://www.acb.org
The council offers a wide variety of services to visually impaired persons with
emphasis on employment opportunities. They publish the *Braille Forum*.

American Foundation for the Blind
11 Penn Plaza, Suite 30
New York, NY 10001
(800) 232-5463
(212) 502-7600
www.afbinfo@afb.org
A national nonprofit organization providing both direct and technical assistance services, including guidance and consultation to blind and visually impaired persons and their families, professionals in the field, community agencies, organizations, schools, and corporations. Also serves as a clearinghouse
for information about blindness and promotes the development of educational,
rehabilitation, and social welfare services for the blind and multiply impaired
deaf-blind children and adults.

American Printing House for the Blind, Inc. (APH)
1839 Frankfort Avenue, P.O. Box 6085
Louisville, KY 40206-0085
(502) 895-2405 (in United States) (800) 223-1839 (in Canada)
info@aph.org
www.aph.org
APH manufactures books and magazines in Braille, large type, and recorded
form. They also create educational and daily living aids, such as slates and

styluses, special tape recorders, talking computer products, and much more. APH offers custom production of items in accessible media, such as Braille menus and recorded annual reports.

American Society for Ophthalmologic Nurses
P.O. Box 193030
San Francisco, CA 94119
(415) 561-8513
www.asorn.org
This is the primary association for nurses in the field of ophthalmology that seeks to improve ophthalmic nursing through research, education, and support.

Choice Magazine Listening
(516) 883-8380
This is a free audio anthology that selects and records over 100 leading magazines for people who are blind or visually impaired. Over 8 hours on tape are provided every other month from major periodicals.

ClinicalTrials.gov
www.clinicaltrials.gov
This Web site provides regularly updated information about federally and privately supported clinical research in human volunteers. It provides information about the latest clinical trials for a disease funded by NIH. Many older adults want to know what is happening in the research world related to their disease. By typing "macular degeneration" or "glaucoma" or "cataracts" in the search box, all the current trials are displayed. Other information can be obtained from this site such as what are clinical trials, search engines for reliable health information, and information on genes and genetic conditions.

Department of Veterans Affairs
Blind Rehabilitation Service (117B)
810 Vermont Avenue, NW
Washington, DC 20420
(202) 273-8482
The Service Program provides for a wide variety of medical and health-related services designed to assist blind veterans in maintaining satisfactory adjustments through their changing circumstances of life and advancing years. These services are based on an annual review that assesses physical, psychological, and social health in addition to evaluating any benefits and resources to which the veteran is entitled. To provide these services, the VA utilizes Visual

Impairment Teams, Blind Rehabilitation Outpatient Specialists, and also residential Blind Rehabilitation Centers throughout the country and Puerto Rico.

Descriptive Video Service
(800) 333-1203
This is a national service that makes television broadcasts and movies on video accessible to blind and visually impaired persons. DVS provides narrated descriptions of essential visual elements without interfering with the audio or dialogue of a program or movie. The narration describes visual elements such as actions, settings, body language, and graphics. A monthly guide is available.

Easter Seals Program
(800) 862-1377
A program that provides services by state-licensed occupational therapists that have specialized training and experience with vision loss. These professionals are available to serve throughout the state of Maryland, South Central Pennsylvania, and the Eastern Panhandle of West Virginia. Therapists may assist with reading, cooking, personal care, household chores, and other aspects of life.

Family Caregiver Alliance
690 Market Street, Suite 600
San Francisco, CA 94104
(800) 445-8106
www.caregiver.org
This organization provides a wealth of information on caregiving through programs of education, research, services, and advocacy.

The Foundation Fighting Blindness, Inc.
Executive Plaza I, Suite 800
11350 McCormick Rd.
Hunt Valley, MD 21031-1014
(888) 394-3937
www.blindness.org
This is a national organization that offers information and support for people with all retinal degenerative diseases. Funding for retinal research is provided.

Healthfinder
www.healthfinder.gov
This is a Web site that provides links to consumer information from the U.S. government, its many partner organizations, and other reliable sources. It

can search over 1,000 health and human service topics. This Web site was developed by the U.S. Department of Health and Human Services.

Independent Living Aids, Inc.
27 East Mall
Plainview, NY 11803
(800) 537-2118
www.independentliving.com
This is a product catalog for low-vision appliances and devices. NOIR glasses, magnifiers, and nonoptical aids can be ordered here.

Leader Dogs for the Blind
P.O. Box 5000
Rochester, MN 48308
888-777-5332
http://www.rollanet.org/~rlions/ldog/
An organization that breeds, raises, trains, and places dogs with a legally blind individual. Residential training with the dog and owner occur on the premises.

Library of Congress National Library Service for the Blind and Physically Handicapped (NLS)
Washington, DC 20542
(202) 707-5100, TDD (202) 707-0744
fax (202) 707-0712
e-mail nl@loc.gov
http://lcweb.loc.gov/nls/
This national organization not only provides books and magazines on tape for blind and physically handicapped individuals but also provides a wealth of information services. Questions on various aspects of blindness and physical disabilities may be sent to the NLS or to any network library. This service is available without charge to individuals, organizations, and libraries. Publications of interest to those people with disabilities and to service providers are free on request. One reference of interest is Blindness and Visual Impairments: Information and Advocacy Organizations, January 1996, No. 96-01. This brochure provides a listing of national and international organizations, agencies, state agencies, and services for the blind and individuals with low vision.

The Lighthouse Inc.
111 East 59th Street
New York, NY 10022

(800) 334-5497

www.lighthouse.org

This nonprofit organization's mission is to "overcome vision impairment for people of all ages through worldwide leadership in rehabilitation services, education, research and advocacy." A large-print newsletter, *Sharing Solutions*, and a catalog of merchandise for those with vision impairment are available.

Low-Vision Electronic Equipment and Computer Software Companies

- Ai Squared
  P.O. Box 669
  Manchester Center, VT 05255
  (800) 859-0270
  http://www.aisquared.com/index.htm
  Makers of *Zoomtext* and *Big Shot*, which are computer programs that provide large print, color contrast, and reading of information on the computer screen. These programs are especially helpful for e-mail and surfing the Internet.

- Artic Technologies
  1000 John R. Road, Suite 108
  Troy, MI 48083
  (248) 588-7370
  www.artictech.com
  This company has many options for magnifiers, portable electronic devices, and note takers.

- Pulse Data HumanWare
  175 Mason Circle
  Concord, CA 94520
  www.pulsedata.com
  (800) 722-3393
  A software company that specializes in personal information management for the low-vision client.

- Telesensory Corporation
  520 Almanor Avenue
  Sunnyvale, CA 94085
  (408) 616-8700
  fax (408) 616-8720
  www.telesensory.com
  This corporation specializes in technology-based products for the low-vision client.

The Macular Degeneration Partnership
www.amd.org
This Web site features a monthly newsletter describing AMD research and publications. The newsletter consists of three parts: (a) Focus on AMD (with contributions from experts in the field of ophthalmology, nutrition, optometry, etc.), (b) The Macular Generation (profiles a patient with macular degeneration each month), and (c) AMD News Update. The site includes information about the disease, controllable and uncontrollable risk factors, active clinical trials for AMD, and information about getting evaluated for the disease. The "Resources" section includes a glossary of terms related to AMD, informative book reviews, and related links on low vision and macular degeneration.

Macular Degeneration Support
www.mdsupport.org
This Web site is designed for user-friendly navigation through topics related to age-related macular degeneration such as diagnosis, treatment, clinical and basic research, education, referral, online chat rooms, and patient stories. An extensive listing of videos, books, and reference material that are available at no cost and for purchase is included.

Maxiaids, Inc.
42 Executive Blvd
Farmingdale, NY 11735
(800) 522-6294
www.maxiaids.com
A low-vision device catalog with numerous options for aids for daily living.

National Alliance for Caregiving
4720 Montgomery Lane, Suite 642
Bethesda, MD 20814
www.caregiving.org
This organization provides reports and fact sheets, holds conferences, and legislates for the needs of professionals and the families that care for an ill family member.

The National Association for the Visually Handicapped (NAVH)
22 West 21st Street 6th Floor
New York, NY 10010
(212) 889-3141
www.navh.org

The mission of this organization is to provide aids, services, and support to the visually impaired. The NAVH site includes a "Low Vision Aids Store" where products can be obtained either online or by phone. The association writes a quarterly newsletter in large print and can be ordered via e-mail or in paper form to your mailbox. It deals with such topics as updates on the Web, new devices to aid vision, and the new $50 bill.

National Eye Health Education Program of the National Eye Institute
2020 Vision Place
Bethesda, MD 20892
(301) 496-5248
(800) 869-2020
www.nei.nih.gov
Provides information on eye problems and vision.

National Federation of the Blind (NFB)
1800 Johnson Street
Baltimore, MD 21230
(410) 659-9314
http://www.nfb.org/
This is a national consumer advocacy organization designed to raise awareness of the needs of the blind and visually impaired. Special services of the NFB include job opportunities for the blind as well as a materials center containing over 1,100 pieces of literature about blindness and 400 different low-vision aids and appliances. In addition, the International Braille and Technology Center for the Blind is the world's largest and most complete evaluation and demonstration center for speech and Braille technology used by the blind from around the world. Newsline® for the Blind, the world's first free talking newspaper service, offers the blind a complete text of leading national and local newspapers with the use of a touch-tone telephone.

New Horizons: Information for the Air Traveler With a Disability
Consumer Information Center
P.O. Box 100
Pueblo, CO 81002
www.dot.gov/airconsumer/horizons.htm
Has a free booklet on consumer rights while flying.

The New York Times Large Type Weekly
P.O. Box 9564
Uniondale, NY 11555-9564

(800) 631-2580
Obtain the week's news in a 40- to 50-page issue with font size 2.5 larger than regular type font. Cost is $1.50 per week.

Recording for the Blind and Dyslexic—Headquarters
The Anne T. MacDonald Center
20 Roszel Road
Princeton, NJ 08540
(800) 221-4792
(609) 452-0606
http://www.rfbd.org
Free cassette tapes, textbooks for students, and materials needed for occupational pursuits are available.

Resources for Rehabilitation
33 Bedford Street, Suite 19A
Lexington, MA 02173
(781) 862-6455
info@rfr.org
www.rfr.org
Training programs for use by the public and professionals on coping with low vision are offered. Materials on coping with low vision are distributed.

The Seeing Eye, Inc.
P.O. Box 375
Morristown, NJ 07963-0375
(973) 539-4425
www.seeingeye.org
The Seeing Eye is a philanthropy that helps people who are blind or visually impaired achieve increased independence and mobility through the use of Seeing Eye dogs. In addition, education and information to the public about the role of dog guides and the capabilities of people who are blind or visually impaired for independent living are provided.

SeniorNet
121 Second St., 7th Floor
San Francisco, CA 94105
(415) 495-4990
http://www.seniornet.org/
A nonprofit organization that provides older adults with education and access to computer technology and the Internet. SeniorNet teaches seniors

(age 50 plus) to use computers and the Internet at over 140 Learning Centers nationwide.

VisionConnection
http://www.visionconnection.org/
A user-friendly Web site founded by Lighthouse International, for all people who have any degree of vision impairment and their families, as well as eye care and low-vision specialists. This site has up-to-date information on most common eye diseases, healthy living to benefit the eyes, and vision rehabilitation. Vision Connection addresses many issues of low vision and readers, and new materials are added weekly.

VISION Foundation, Inc.
818 Mt. Auburn Street
Watertown, MA 02172
(617) 926-4232
(617) 926-0289 voice/TDD
(800) 852-3029 in Massachusetts
Fax: (617) 926-1412
A self-help organization serving persons who are newly born blind, have low vision, or have a progressive eye disease. Support groups, an information and referral center, a buddy telephone system, a career mentor program, special programs for older people, and materials in large print or cassette are offered.

Voice Activated Dialing From Verizon
(800) 870-0000
Automatic dialing can be obtained by programming the older adult's voice into his or her phone. This program can store up to 50 names per household.

Booklets

What You Should Know About Low Vision
(301) 496-5248
http://www.nei.nih.gov/
A free large-print booklet published by the National Eye Institute that can assist people to understand low vision and what can be done for it. It provides suggestions of questions to ask an eye care specialist as well as resources for more information.

When Your Partner Becomes Visually Impaired . . . Helpful Insights and Tips for Coping
by Carol J. Sussman-Skalka, CSW, MBA

(800) 334-5497
The Lighthouse Inc.
111 East 59th Street
New York, NY 10022
A free, large-print booklet that describes specific concerns of the spouse of someone diagnosed with a visual impairment. Understanding the partner, improving communications, taking advantage of resources, and handling stress are some of the topics covered in this booklet.

Federal Programs for Financial Assistance

Property Tax
In many states, any legally blind person who owns and resides in his or her home as well as the surviving spouse of a legally blind resident may qualify for a reduction of the assessed value of the real estate. A certain amount of the assessed value is disregarded when calculating the property tax. The State Department of Assessment and Taxation should be contacted for more information.

Social Security Disability Insurance (SSDI)
Visually handicapped individuals may be eligible for Social Security benefits. Benefits are based on how much a worker has paid into the Social Security fund through payroll deduction, not on financial need. Family income and assets are not counted in determining the benefits. After receiving disability for 2 years, a disabled person will also be protected under Medicare, the federal health insurance program.

Supplemental Security Income (SSI)
People who are legally blind with little or no regular income, savings or assets, may be eligible for monthly income through SSI. Financial need is considered in determining eligibility benefits. Benefits may be received even if the recipient has never been employed. In most states, people receiving SSI are also eligible for Medical Assistance (Medicaid).

For more information on SSI & SSDI, the Social Security Administration in MD: (800) 772-1213 or The National Federation of the Blind: (410) 659–9314 may be contacted.

Tax Exemptions
Any legally blind taxpayer may obtain an extra exemption on both state and federal tax returns. This means that a person's gross income may be reduced by the amount of the exemption when calculating taxes. When submitting a tax return, a copy of the letter written by the physician stating that the person

is legally blind should be attached to the return. Contact the Internal Revenue Service: (800) 829-1040.

Religious Programs

Aurora Ministries
P.O. Box 621
Bradenton, FL 34206
(914) 748-4100
Aurora Ministries provide Bible cassette tapes free to the visually impaired of the world. The New Testament is available in 55 languages. Verification of impairment is required. Complimentary sets are provided for doctors, organizations, and care professionals working with the visually impaired.

John Milton Society for the Blind
475 Riverside Drive, Room 455
New York, NY 10115
(212) 870-3335
Provides free Christian literature in Braille, audiocassettes, and large type.

The Jewish Braille Institute of America
(800) 433-1531
www.jewishbraille.org
An institute that offers many books of interest on audiocassette, Braille, and large print. Materials are available to anyone who is blind, visually impaired, or physically or learning disabled. Services and materials are free of charge.

The Xavier Society for the Blind
(212) 473-7800
Mass texts, audiocassette Bibles, the Catechism of the Catholic Church, and a wealth of other materials are available in large print or in audiotapes for no charge.

Recommended Reading for Older Adults With Low Vision and Their Families

Cassel, G., Billig, M., & Randall, H. (1998). *The eye book: A complete guide to eye disorders and health.* Baltimore: Johns Hopkins Press Health Book.

D'Amato, R., & Snyder, J (2000). *Macular degeneration: The latest scientific discoveries and treatments for preserving your sight.* New York: Walker & Co.

Grunwald, H. (1999). *Twilight, losing sight, gaining insight.* New York: Alfred A. Knopf.

Mogk, L., & Mogk, M. (2003). *Macular degeneration: The complete guide to saving and maximizing your sight.* New York: Ballantine Books.

Peli, E., & Peli, D. (2002). *Driving with confidence: A practical guide to driving with low vision.* London: World Scientific Publishing Company, Pte. Ltd.

Rosenthal, B., & Kelly, K. (2001). *Living well with macular degeneration.* New York: New American Library.

Solomon, Y. (2000). *Overcoming macular degeneration—A guide to seeing beyond the clouds.* New York: Avon Books, Inc.

REFERENCES

Brody, B. L., Roch-Levecq, A.-C., Gamst, A. C., Maclean, K., Kaplan, R. M., & Brown, S. I. (2002). Self-management of age-related macular degeneration and quality of life. *Archives of Ophthalmology, 120,* 1477–1483.

Dahlin-Ivanoff, S., Klepp, K. I., & Sjostrand, J. (1998). Development of a health education programme for elderly with age-related macular degeneration: A focus group study. *Patient Education and Counseling, 34*(1), 63–73.

Davison, K., Pennebaker, J., & Dickerson, S. (2000). Who talks? The social psychology of illness support groups. *American Psychologist, 55*(2), 205–217.

Deremerick, J. (2003). New low vision technology. *MacFacts, 5,* 6.

Fletcher, D. (1994). Low vision: The physician's role in rehabilitation and referral. *Geriatrics, 49*(5), 50–54.

Gieser, J. P. (2004). When treatment fails: Caring for patients with visual disability. *Archives of Ophthalmology, 122*(8), 1208–1209.

Greenblatt, S. L. (1989). *Providing services for people with vision loss.* Lexington, MA: Resources for Rehabilitation.

Hinds, A., Sinclair, A., Park, J., Suttie, A., Paterson, H., & Macdonald, M. (2003). Impact of an interdisciplinary low vision service on the quality of life of low vision patients. *British Journal of Ophthalmology, 87*(11), 1391–1396.

Kupfer, C. (2000). The National Eye Institute's Low Vision Education Program: Improving quality of life. *Ophthalmology, 107*(2), 229–230.

Margrain, T. H. (2000). Helping blind and partially sighted people to read: The effectiveness of low vision aids. *British Journal of Ophthalmology, 84*(8), 919–921.

Rovner, B. W., & Casten, R. J. (2002). Activity loss and depression in age-related macular degeneration. *American Journal of Geriatric Psychiatry, 10,* 305–310.

Rovner, B. W., Casten, R. J., & Tasman, W. (2002). Effect of depression on vision function in age-related macular degeneration. *Archives of Ophthalmology, 120*(8), 1041–1044.

Schuchard, R. (1999). Characteristics of AMD patients with low vision receiving visual rehabilitation. *Journal of Rehabilitation Research and Development, 36*(4), 294–302.

Scott, I. U., Smiddy, W. E., Schiffman, J., Feuer, W. J., & Pappas, C. J. (1999). Quality of life of low-vision patients and the impact of low-vision services. *American Journal of Ophthalmology, 128*(1), 54–62.

Stelmack, J. (2001). Quality of life of low-vision patients and outcomes of low-vision rehabilitation. *Optometry and Vision Science, 78*(5), 335–342.

The Eye Diseases Prevalence Research Group. (2004). Causes and prevalence of visual impairment among adults in the United States. *Archives of Ophthalmology, 122*(4), 477–485.

Watson, G. R. (2001). Low vision in the geriatric population: Rehabilitation and management. *Journal of the American Geriatrics Society, 49*(3), 317–330.

CHAPTER 11

Future Directions in the Care of Older Adults With Age-Related Vision Loss

Kate Goldblum, Pat Gillett, and Joyce Powers

AGE-RELATED MACULAR DEGENERATION

The leading cause of blindness in the United States is age-related macular degeneration (AMD) with 1.75 million individuals affected by a significant central loss of vision, most due to choroidal neovascularization (Ho et al., 2004). The trend toward an increasingly aged population suggests that the impact of this problem will increase greatly over the next several decades. Up to 3 million individuals will be impacted (Eye Diseases Prevalence Research Group, 2004). Less visually significant AMD affects even greater numbers—up to 7 million individuals may have intermediate AMD (Preferred Practice Patterns Committee [PPPC], Retina Panel, 2003a). Although there is significant ongoing research into treatments for both nonexudative (dry or atrophic) and exudative (wet) AMD, preventing progression to advanced AMD is currently the best strategy to reduce the impact of this devastating condition (Bressler, 2004).

Recent Developments in Treatment

Although there is currently no known means to prevent AMD, recent research into treatments preventing the progression of vision loss from AMD is encouraging and provides additional hope for the future. Results to date of a randomized, placebo-controlled, clinical trial provide evidence that the combination of antioxidant vitamins and minerals reduced vision loss progression.

This was true only in patients classified as having intermediate or advanced nonexudative AMD, not in those patients with milder forms of the disorder (Age-Related Eye Disease Study [AREDS] Research Group, 2001a). One of the classification criteria used by the AREDS Research Group included the presence and extent of drusens, which are yellowish hyaline deposits under the retinal pigment epithelium. Due to the number of individuals with intermediate or advanced AMD, supplement use would have a significant public health impact in the United States (AREDS Research Group, 2003).

There is also current evidence to support other "state-of-the-art" therapies for AMD, including thermal laser photocoagulation and photodynamic therapy (PDT). Research supports the efficacy of thermal laser photocoagulation for patients with well-defined neovascular lesions that are at least 200 microns from the center of the fovea (juxtafoveal) or between 1 and 199 microns from the center of the fovea (extrafoveal). Treating patients with lesions directly under the foveal center (subfoveal) produces an immediate loss of some central vision. However, those patients, even with immediate vision loss, retained more vision than did untreated patients after 2 years (Macular Photocoagulation Study Group [MPSG], 1991, 1993, 1994). Patients and families must understand this problematic issue and be willing to accept immediate and permanent loss of some vision following a treatment that will provide a future benefit. Thermal laser is not the first choice for initial treatment in patients with subfoveal lesions (PPPC, Retina Panel, 2003a).

Photodynamic therapy (PDT) using the light-activated drug, verteporfin (Visudyne) has proven to be valuable in arresting progression of vision loss in individuals with subfoveal, exudative AMD (Treatment of Age-Related Macular Degeneration With Photodynamic Therapy [TAP] Study Group, 1999, 2001, 2002; TAP and Verteporfin Photodynamic Therapy [VIP] Study Groups, 2003). These studies are ongoing. They seek to further identify the beneficial aspects of PDT, compare its effectiveness to other therapies, and explore the potential synergistic effect when combined with other therapies. Although patients treated with PDT cannot expect vision improvement, they may experience less progression of vision loss following treatment. Other problematic issues include the need for re-treatments and the potential complications, including extravasation of verteporfin at the infusion site, photosensitivity reactions, and back pain during infusion.

Therapeutic Options for the Future

Many other promising or potential therapies for AMD are currently under study (Ho et al., 2004). None currently have enough research support to allow clear recommendations for using them (PPPC, Retina Panel, 2003a). Several ongoing studies of choroidal neovascularization (CNV) prevention with prophylactic laser in patients with drusen have shown promise (Weissgold & Fardin, 2003a). Dietary supplementation with antioxidant micronutrients other than those in the AREDS formulation may also be beneficial. These include lutein, zeaxanthin, bilberry, and gingko biloba. Lutein, 6 mg/day, and zeaxanthin, 1,000 μg/day, are probably safe, but there is no conclusive evidence that they are helpful. Bilberry and gingko biloba both increase retinal blood flow and exhibit antioxidant activity, but lack of therapeutic trials limits knowledge about the clinical effects of these herbal supplements (Weissgold & Fardin, 2003a). Further research may clarify the potential role of these and other micronutrients in preventing or treating nonexudative AMD.

Several surgical options for exudative AMD are under study. With submacular surgery and pneumatic displacement, the surgical rationale is to remove subfoveal CNV or blood. With macular translocation, the surgical rationale is to move the macula to an area of undamaged retina. Another treatment option is radiation therapy in low doses, which may slow the growth of new vessels. Transpupillary thermotherapy may also slow neovascularization as well as occlude those already present (Weissgold & Fardin, 2003b). Angiostatic steroids, alone or in combination with PDT, also inhibit angiogenesis and researchers are continuing to study their use in patients with CNV. Anecortave acetate (Retaane), a newer intravitreal angiostatic steroid with no corticosteroid activity, is also currently under study. It is less likely than the corticosteroids to produce intraocular pressure increase and cataract formation (Singerman, 2004). Antivascular endothelial growth factor (VEGF) compounds also inhibit angiogenesis. Pegaptanib sodium (Macugen) and ranibizumab (Lucentis) are currently in late stage clinical trials.

Gene therapy is a potentially promising development, although its use for patients with AMD is many years away. Other treatments aimed at replacing damaged photoreceptor cells in nonexudative AMD include retinal implants and transplant of retinal pigment epithelium or photoreceptor cells. Applying these procedures in patients with AMD is probably decades in the future (Weissgold & Fardin, 2003a).

Nursing Implications

The increase in numbers of patients with AMD predicted for the future will necessitate a team approach. Nurses will fill critical roles. They will obtain assessment data based on focused patient histories, provide patient education, and make referrals to appropriate resources. Referral to an ophthalmologist will be urgent for patients with AMD who may present with blurred vision unexplained by other obvious causes or new metamorphopsia, a visual defect in which patients perceive objects as distorted in shape. In addition, any patients in whom funduscopic examination reveals hard exudates or hemorrhages in the retina will need urgent referral to assure appropriate and timely assessment and treatment.

Patients with AMD often have significant knowledge deficits. Nurses are uniquely suited to provide accurate and timely patient education as well as emotional support. Nurses' holistic approach will be absolutely critical in caring for patients with AMD. Depression is a common and understandable response to vision loss and can contribute to patients' perceptions of a decline in visual function, even when there has been no actual change in visual acuity (Rovner, Casten, & Tasman, 2002). Nurses will help identify patients who are, or may be, depressed. They will also provide appropriate nursing care, including facilitating referrals to mental health care professionals for additional care. Advanced practice nurses will be involved in treating patients' depression.

Patients with AMD will also need information on disease process, prognosis, treatment options, or community and other resources for vision rehabilitation and socioeconomic support. The large numbers of patients with AMD projected for the future will necessitate an efficient and effective process to provide this information. Nurses should develop a file of national and local resources for easy access and dissemination to patients and their families. Emotional support is critical for patients who have loss of vision and face potential blindness. Realistic encouragement will be appropriate in most cases, and nurses will need to stay abreast of new developments in therapeutic options for AMD in order to provide the most current and accurate information. Even when treatment fails to improve vision or arrest progressive vision loss, patients will find comfort in understanding that "blindness" from AMD does not mean total blackness. Using their intact peripheral vision can provide significant benefit. It is imperative that these patients are not told "there is nothing else we can do" if they have AMD with vision loss. The many current and future options for therapy or low-vision rehabilitation can help them maintain an active and vital lifestyle.

CATARACTS

Cataracts of varying significance are a common condition in older adults, becoming almost ubiquitous in the very old. In those over age 75, visually significant cataracts occur in almost 40% of men and 46% of women. In the United States, cataract is the leading cause of reversible blindness in individuals over age 40, whereas worldwide, it is the leading cause of blindness in all individuals (PPPC, Anterior Segment Panel, 2001). As the population ages, the numbers of affected individuals will increase, making cataract a significant quality of life issue.

Recent Developments in Treatment

Cataract prevention is obviously preferable to treatment. Research has implicated many risk factors for cataract development, some of which are potentially modifiable (PPPC, Anterior Segment Panel, 2001; Solomon & Donnenfeld, 2003). To the extent that patients may be able to control or modify those risk factors, it may be possible to decrease the risk of cataract development or progression. Unfortunately, no well-controlled studies to date provide support for any preventive strategy, including nutritional supplementation with vitamins or minerals (AREDS Research Group, 2001b). There is also no evidence that any nonsurgical method can eliminate cataracts or slow their development (PPPC, Anterior Segment Panel). In recent years, however, surgical treatment has greatly improved. Ophthalmologists now remove cataracts primarily under topical anesthesia and patients usually require only a few hours' stay in an outpatient surgical facility. Foldable intraocular lenses and ultrasonic fragmentation of the lens allow small incisions, rapid recovery, and almost immediate visual rehabilitation.

Therapeutic Options for the Future

Continued research into better methods of lens fragmentation will lead to fewer potential problems from the heat and cavitation that result from ultrasonic phacoemulsification of cataracts. Improved intraocular lens designs will allow even smaller incisions. Improvement of current multifocal designs will give better quality vision while still giving patients the ability to see clearly at distance and near. New laser technology should increase the precision of axial length measurements, allowing greater accuracy in calculating intraocular lens power (Woodcock, Shad, & Smith, 2004). This would result in optimal vision without additional spectacle correction for greater numbers of patients after surgery.

Nursing Implications

Increasing numbers of older individuals will impact the numbers of cataract surgeries performed in the future. In 1999, Medicare patients not enrolled in a health maintenance organization had 1.6 million cataract surgeries (PPPC, Anterior Segment Panel, 2001). Given this fact, a huge number of individuals will potentially have cataract surgery.

Although cataract surgery is extremely safe and almost always provides excellent visual outcomes, older adults need to be involved in the decision whether or not to proceed with surgery. The decision-making process should take the individual patient's visual needs into consideration. In most cases, the only indication for cataract surgery is that the patient cannot function adequately and has a reduced quality of life due to reduced vision. The decision-making process can be time consuming, especially in older patients who may require more time to process unfamiliar information. Nurses will be invaluable in helping patients assimilate the information they need to make an appropriately informed decision about cataract surgery.

As this cohort of older patients increases, the number of individuals with comorbidities will also increase, potentially impacting the safety of cataract surgery. Nurses can assess the significance of those co-morbidities and conduct or arrange for further evaluation as appropriate. Assuring that patients arrive for cataract surgery with all necessary assessments completed enhances patients' safety and minimizes last-minute cancellations. This increases surgical facility efficiency and lowers costs—an important consideration with increasingly limited health care resources.

Another issue is that patients who have cataract surgery arrive home only a few hours after the procedure. Although many patients will have adequate health care resources in place, others will not. Their primary needs will be for information and supportive care, not direct physical care. Some facilities or clinics currently have adequate plans for this type of ongoing care, but future needs will demand more nursing involvement. A greater number of nurses from home health care agencies, surgical facilities, offices, and clinics will need to provide postoperative education and support.

GLAUCOMA

Glaucoma is a significant cause of legal blindness in the United States, especially in African American individuals. The most common form of glaucoma, primary open-angle glaucoma (POAG), affects approximately 2.5 million individuals in the United States (PPPC, Glaucoma Panel, 2003). Like systemic hypertension, many people with glaucoma do not know they have the disorder because there are few symptoms to indicate a possible problem. Loss of visual field is only apparent after long-term disease presence.

Recent Developments in Treatment

Ophthalmologists recognize that glaucoma is a complex problem. Although other factors contribute to the loss of retinal cells and optic nerve fibers that eventually causes progressive visual field loss, lowering IOP is the mainstay of treatment (PPPC, Glaucoma Panel, 2003). One challenging problem has been deciding whether and when to treat patients with ocular hypertension, who have increased IOP but no evidence of glaucomatous damage. Recent research has led to the recognition that ocular hypertension, if untreated, will progress to glaucomatous damage within 5 years in 1 out of every 10 patients and that treatment can significantly reduce the onset of glaucoma (Kass et al., 2002). Conversely, about 15% to 40% of patients with IOPs below 21 mm Hg carry a diagnosis of normal-tension glaucoma and exhibit the typical characteristics of POAG (PPPC, Glaucoma Panel). Several recent clinical studies confirmed that IOP plays an important role in progression of glaucomatous damage and provided evidence that lowering IOP from the patient's baseline can ameliorate this progression (Schwartz & Budenz, 2004; Wilson & Brandt, 2003).

Current therapy to lower IOP includes medical therapy, laser procedures, and incisional surgeries. The older pharmacologic agents used to lower IOP are now largely replaced by newer drugs with improved efficacy and better side-effect profiles. These include topical beta-blocking agents, topical carbonic an-hydrase inhibitors, and prostaglandin analogs. Increasingly, ophthalmologists employ lasers in treating glaucoma, but only occasionally as initial therapy (Schwartz & Budenz, 2004). Surgical options are now considered at earlier points in the disease process rather than delaying surgery until other thera-pies have failed (Khaw, Shah, & Elkington, 2004). Newer surgical techniques include implanted aqueous shunts, such as the Molteno implant. This type of surgery provides options in cases where more traditional surgeries to increase aqueous outflow are not likely to be effective (Sidoti & Heuer, 2002).

Therapeutic Options for the Future

One of the most difficult issues surrounding patients with ocular hypertension is when and whether to begin treatment. Similarly, it is currently difficult to know whether treatment will truly benefit patients who do exhibit glauco-matous damage because not all patients actually lose functional vision during their lifetime (Weinreb, 2004). One approach to the problem is to develop a valid risk-assessment model, similar to that applied to managing patients with coronary heart disease. Further research in this area should provide ophthal-mologists with better answers to this important question and lead to analyses of the number-needed-to-treat and treatment cost-effectiveness. Having this information will help ophthalmologists develop strategies for preventing pro-gression from ocular hypertension to glaucoma and guide treatment for those patients with glaucoma (Girkin, Kannel, Friedman, & Weinreb, 2004).

The rationale for lowering IOP is to indirectly protect the optic nerve by reducing the damage caused by ocular hypertension. This rationale is being expanded to include protective efforts that will offer protection directly. Researchers are studying pharmacologic agents that increase blood flow to the optic nerve head and neuroprotective agents that improve optic nerve metabolism or reduce ischemic insult (Kaushik, Pandav, & Ram, 2003). Genetic approaches include testing to help identify patients likely to develop glaucoma and glaucomatous damage and identifying glaucoma genes which could lead to development of pharmacologic agents to directly affect the gene or its products (Samples & Wirtz, 2003). Regeneration of the optic nerve is another approach being studied.

Other developments are helping guide diagnostic and treatment decisions and are the subject of continued research. Improved methods of mapping a patient's visual field will lead to earlier diagnosis and recognition of progressive glaucomatous damage (Greenstein, Thienprasiddhi, Ritch, Liebmann, & Hood, 2004; Johnson, 2002). Tomography may provide better, quantitative information useful in documenting optic disc morphology and observing disease progression (Wilson & Brandt, 2003). Determining corneal thickness is now recognized as an important factor in assessing the significance and specific risk of a patient's IOP, and continued research will help clarify the role of corneal thickness in guiding diagnosis and treatment (Girkin et al., 2004; Wilson & Brandt).

Nursing Implications

As with AMD, glaucoma is a chronic and noncurable, but treatable, disorder. Nurses assess, diagnose, and treat patients' responses to their health problems. Patients with chronic disorders such as glaucoma, in which adherence to therapy is imperative, are particularly appropriate targets for nursing interventions. To provide optimal care to patients with glaucoma, a greater number of ophthalmologists will need to recognize the value of nurses who can provide this type of care and work collaboratively with them, both in ophthalmic practice settings and in primary care. Nurses offer a unique perspective on care for patients with chronic, treatable disorders such as glaucoma.

DIABETIC RETINOPATHY

The duration of diabetes is closely related to development of diabetic retinopathy. Nearly all patients with diabetes will eventually develop diabetic retinopathy of some degree. After 15 years of disease presence, 80% of patients with type 1 diabetes mellitus will have retinopathy. In type 2 disease, duration of up to 19 years is associated with retinopathy in 84% of those patients using insulin and 53% of those not using insulin (PPPC, Retina Panel, 2003b). With increasing numbers of individuals in the United States diagnosed with diabetes, many more older Americans will have diabetic retinopathy in the future.

Recent Developments in Treatment

Current recommended treatment strategies are 90% effective in preventing severe vision loss secondary to diabetic retinopathy (PPPC, Retina Panel, 2003b). Timely focal and pan-retinal lasers are accepted modalities that can help maintain good visual acuity in most patients (Chew et al., 2003). The Diabetes Control and Complications Trial (DCCT) showed that strict glycemic control delayed onset and progression of diabetic retinopathy in patients with type 1 diabetes (The DCCT Research Group, 1993). A similar study of patients with type 2 diabetes also provided support for the value of intensive control of blood glucose levels in preventing the microvascular complications of diabetes (The United Kingdom Prospective Diabetes Study [UKPDS] Group, 1998). Recognition that control of systemic hypertension and serum cholesterol levels also contributes to prevention of complications has led to clinical application of the diabetic "ABCs": hemoglobin A_{1c}, **B**lood pressure, and **C**holesterol (The United Kingdom Prospective Diabetes Study Group, 2004). Teaching the "ABCs" of diabetes is a way to educate patients on the importance of these factors in preventing diabetic complications, including vision loss.

Therapeutic Options for the Future

The association of vascular endothelial cell growth factor (VEGF) with development of neovascularization and macular edema in patients with diabetes points to the fact that research into pharmacologic and other modalities to inhibit VEGF (discussed earlier in this chapter under age-related macular degeneration) may also prove beneficial in these patients (Fong & Ferris, 2003). Additional research could also clarify the roles of other factors in preventing development and progression of diabetic retinopathy and macular edema and of newer treatment modalities (Christoforidis & D'Amico, 2004).

Nursing Implications

Vision loss secondary to diabetic retinopathy might be expected to increase greatly in the future given the increasing number of people being diagnosed with diabetes. It is largely preventable, however, and nurses will have an important role in this prevention. With their broad-based education in health care and expertise in patient education, nurses are going to be critically important in helping patients understand the importance of controlling not only blood glucose levels but also blood pressure, cholesterol, and other systemic factors. Nurses will also be crucial in helping patients manage the difficulties of adhering to complex insulin and other treatment regimens. Nurses in ophthalmology and primary care settings will have opportunities to assist in providing direct care, coordinating care among patients' various providers, promoting recommended follow-up, and supporting those patients who do sustain severe loss despite treatment.

SUMMARY

Nurses will play a major role in caring for patients with actual or potential age-related vision loss in the future. Nurses often have significant and important research roles as well. Future research in the area of age-related vision loss is focusing on exciting and innovative preventive and treatment modalities. Nurses' holistic framework will be invaluable in research roles, as well as in the many other ways in which nurses care for patients with macular degeneration, cataracts, glaucoma, and diabetic retinopathy.

REFERENCES

Age-Related Eye Disease Study Research Group. (2001a). A randomized, placebo-controlled, clinical trial of high-dose supplementation with vitamins C and E and beta carotene for age-related macular degeneration and vision loss: AREDS report no. 8. *Archives of Ophthalmology, 119*, 1417–1436.

Age-Related Eye Disease Study Research Group. (2001b). A randomized, placebo-controlled, clinical trial of high-dose supplementation with vitamins C and E and beta carotene for age-related cataract and vision loss: AREDS report no. 9. *Archives of Ophthalmology, 119*, 1439–1452.

Age-Related Eye Disease Study Research Group. (2003). Potential public health impact of AREDS results: AREDS report no. 11. *Archives of Ophthalmology, 121*, 1621–1624.

Bressler, N. M. (2004). Age-related macular degeneration is the leading cause of blindness. *JAMA, 291*(15), 1900–1901.

Chew, E. Y., Ferris, F. L., Csaky, K G., Murphy, R. P, Agrón, E., Thompson, D. J. S., Reed, G. F., & Schachat, A. P. (2003). The long-term effects of laser photocoagulation treatment in patients with diabetic retinopathy: The Early Treatment Diabetic Retinopathy Follow-up Study. *Ophthalmology, 110*(9), 1683–1689.

Christoforidis, J. B., & D'Amico, D. J. (2004). Surgical and other treatments of diabetic macular edema: An update. *International Ophthalmology Clinics, 44*(1), 139–160.

Eye Diseases Prevalence Research Group. (2004). Prevalence of age-related macular degeneration in the United States. *Archives of Ophthalmology, 122*, 564–572.

Fong, D. S., & Ferris, F. L. (2003). Practical management of diabetic retinopathy. *Focal Points, XXI*(3), 1–18. San Francisco: American Academy of Ophthalmology.

Girkin, C. A., Kannel, W. B., Friedman, D. S., & Weinreb, R. N. (2004). Glaucoma risk factor assessment and prevention: Lessons from coronary heart disease. *American Journal of Ophthalmology, 138*(3, Suppl.), S11–S18.

Greenstein, V. C., Thienprasiddhi, P., Ritch, R., Liebmann, J. M., & Hood, D. C. (2004). A method for comparing electrophysiological, psychophysical, and structural measures of glaucomatous damage. *Archives of Ophthalmology, 122*(9), 1276–1284.

Ho, A. C., Brucker, A. J., Ferris, F. L., Kaiser, P. K., Regillo, C. D., Slakter, J. S., Spaide, R., Thomas, M. A., & Vander, J. F. (2004, October 24). *New and investigational therapies for age-related macular degeneration.* Course presented at the annual meeting of the American Academy of Ophthalmology in New Orleans.

Johnson, C. A. (2002). Recent development in automated perimetry in glaucoma diagnosis and management. *Current Opinion in Ophthalmology, 13*(1), 77–84.

Kass, M. A., Heuer, D. K., Higginbotham, E. J., Johnson, C. A., Keltner, J. L., Miller, J. P., Parrish, R. K., 2nd, Wilson, M. R., & Gordon, M. O. (2002). The ocular hypertension treatment study: A randomized trial determines that topical ocular hypotensive medication delays or prevents the onset of primary open angle glaucoma. *Archives of Ophthalmology, 120*, 701–713.

Kaushik, S., Pandav, S. S., & Ram, J. (2003). Neuroprotection in glaucoma. *Journal of Postgraduate Medicine, 49*(1), 90–95.

Khaw, P. T., Shah, P., & Elkington, A. R. (2004). Glaucoma—2: Treatment. *British Medical Journal, 328*, 156–158.

Macular Photocoagulation Study Group. (1991). Argon laser photocoagulation for neovascular maculopathy. Five-year results from randomized clinical trials. *Archives of Ophthalmology, 109*, 1109–1114.

Macular Photocoagulation Study Group. (1993). Laser photocoagulation of subfoveal neovascular lesions of age-related macular degeneration. Updated findings from two clinical trials. *Archives of Ophthalmology, 111*, 1200–1209.

Macular Photocoagulation Study Group. (1994). Laser photocoagulation for juxtafoveal choroidal neovascularization. Five-year results from randomized clinical trials. *Archives of Ophthalmology, 112*, 500–509.

Preferred Practice Patterns Committee, Anterior Segment Panel. (2001). *Preferred practice pattern: Cataract in the adult eye.* San Francisco: American Academy of Ophthalmology.

Preferred Practice Patterns Committee, Glaucoma Panel. (2003). *Preferred practice pattern: Primary open-angle glaucoma.* San Francisco: American Academy of Ophthalmology.

Preferred Practice Patterns Committee, Retina Panel. (2003a). *Preferred practice pattern: Age-related macular degeneration.* San Francisco: American Academy of Ophthalmology.

Preferred Practice Patterns Committee, Retina Panel. (2003b). *Preferred practice pattern: Diabetic retinopathy*. San Francisco: American Academy of Ophthalmology.

Rovner, B. W., Casten, R. J., & Tasman, W. S. (2002). Effect of depression on vision function in age-related macular degeneration. *Archives of Ophthalmology, 120*, 1041–1044.

Samples, J. R., & Wirtz, M. K. (2003). Introductory ophthalmic genetics. *Ophthalmology Clinics of North America, 16*(4), 501–503.

Schwartz, K., & Budenz, D. (2004). Current management of glaucoma. *Current Opinion in Ophthalmology, 15*(2), 119–126.

Sidoti, P. A., & Heuer, D. K. (2002). *Aqueous shunting procedures. Focal Points, XX*(3), 1–14. San Francisco: American Academy of Ophthalmology.

Singerman, L. J. (2004). A clinician's guide to retinal disease: Pharmacology for age-related macular degeneration. *Review of Ophthalmology, Part 2 of 2, September* 12–15.

Solomon, R., & Donnenfeld, E. D. (2003). Recent advances and future frontiers in treating age-related cataracts. *JAMA, 290*(2), 248–251.

The Diabetes Control and Complications Research Group. (1993). The effect of intensive treatment of diabetes on the development and progression of long-term complications in insulin-dependent diabetes mellitus. *New England Journal of Medicine, 329*, 977–986.

The United Kingdom Prospective Diabetes Study Group. (1998). Effect of intensive blood-glucose control with metformin on complications in overweight patients with type 2 diabetes (UKPDS 34). *Lancet, 352*, 854–865.

The United Kingdom Prospective Diabetes Study Group. (2004). Risk of progression of retinopathy and vision loss related to tight blood pressure control in Type 2 diabetes mellitus. *Archives of Ophthalmology, 122*, 1631–1640.

Treatment of Age-Related Macular Degeneration with Photodynamic Therapy (TAP) Study Group. (1999). Photodynamic therapy of subfoveal choroidal neovascularization in age-related macular degeneration with verteporfin: One year results of 2 randomized clinical trials—TAP report 1. *Archives of Ophthalmology, 117*, 1329–1345.

Treatment of Age-Related Macular Degeneration with Photodynamic Therapy (TAP) Study Group. (2001). Photodynamic therapy of subfoveal choroidal neovascularization in age-related macular degeneration with verteporfin: Two-year results of 2 randomized clinical trials—TAP report 2. *Archives of Ophthalmology, 119*, 198–207.

Treatment of Age-Related Macular Degeneration with Photodynamic Therapy (TAP) Study Group. (2002). Verteporfin therapy for subfoveal choroidal neovascularization in age-related macular degeneration: Three-year results of an open-label extension of 2 randomized clinical trials—TAP report no. 5. *Archives of Ophthalmology, 120*, 1307–1314.

Treatment of Age-Related Macular Degeneration with Photodynamic Therapy (TAP) and Verteporfin in Photodynamic Therapy (VIP) Study Groups. (2003). Photodynamic therapy of subfoveal choroidal neovascularization with verteporfin:

Fluorescein angiographic guidelines for evaluation and treatment—TAP and VIP report no. 2. *Archives of Ophthalmology, 121*, 1253–1268.

Weinreb, R. N. (2004). Ocular hypertension: Defining risks and clinical options. *American Journal of Ophthalmology, 138*(3, supplement), S1-S-2.

Weissgold, D. J., & Fardin, B. (2003a). Advances in the treatment of nonexudative age-related macular degeneration. *Focal Points, XXI*(5), 1–14. San Francisco: American Academy of Ophthalmology.

Weissgold, D. J., & Fardin, B. (2003b). Advances in the treatment of exudative age-related macular degeneration. *Focal Points, XXI*(6), 1–16. San Francisco: American Academy of Ophthalmology.

Wilson, M. R., & Brandt, J.D. (2003). Update of glaucoma clinical trials. *Focal Points, XXI*(9), 1–14. San Francisco: American Academy of Ophthalmology.

Woodcock, M., Shad, S., & Smith, R. J. (2004). Recent advances in customising cataract surgery. *British Medical Journal, 328*, 92–96.

Index

Note: An f after a page number indicates a figure; a t after a page number indicates a table

eye examinations
for AMD, 21, 22
for diabetic retinopathy, 65, 69, 70
for glaucoma, 51–54
of pupil, 31
eyelids, drooping of, 6–7

families
education's importance to, 152–153
health of/evaluation process of, 156–157
help possibilities of, 152–154
intervention planning for, 153–154
lack of awareness/relatability within,
150–151
as part of treatment team, 152
support groups for, 153
Family Caregiver Alliance, 178
fat, AMD influenced by, 96–97
Federal Programs for Financial Assistance
property tax, 185–186
Social Security Disability Insurance, 185
Supplemental Security Income, 185
tax exemptions, 185
Ferris-Bailey Chart assessment, 133
fields of vision assessment, 135
fish intake, AMD influenced by, 96–97
fluorescein scan, 77
focal laser, 84f
focal photocoagulation surgery, 82–84
Folkman, S., 113
Foundation Fighting Blindness, Inc.,
178
functional independence
importance of, 121
potential losses of, 123

gene therapy, 191
glare
cataracts and, 32
decreasing tolerance to, 5
glasses, for reading, 6
glaucoma
African Americans and, 41, 98
alpha$_2$-adrenergic agonists for, 58t
angle-closure glaucoma, 42
gender preference, 44
risks of, 44
symptoms, 45
visual field defects, 42–43
beta-blockers for, 47t
brimonidine tartrate for, 58t
carbonic anhydrase inhibitors (CAIs) for,
48t
cigarette smoking as risk factor, 97
combination agents for, 59t
dorcolamide 2% timolol maleate for, 59t
early detection procedures, 45–46,
49–54

eye examination
anterior chamber assessment, 52–53
color vision assessment, 51
external structures assessment, 53
extraocular muscle tests, 51–52
general survey, 50
internal structures assessment, 53–54
IOP measurement, 54
pupils/pupillary reflex assessment, 52
visual acuity tests, 50
visual fields assessment, 51
focused health history of older adults, 46,
49–50
future therapeutic options, 195–196
IOP in, 42
laser procedures for, 55, 60
latanoprost for, 57t
medical management of, 55, 60
miotics for, 56t
narrow-angle, 70
nurse's role in treatment of, 60–62
nursing implications, 195–196, 196
open-angle glaucoma, 41, 42
as asymptomatic, 44–45
causes of, 43
racial preference, 44
visual field defects, 42–43
pathophysiology/risk factors of, 43–44
phacomorphic, 31–32
prevention of, 97–98
prostaglandin analogs for, 57t
racial preference of, 41
recent treatment developments, 194–195
scotoma and, 42–43
as second leading cause of blindness, 9–10,
41
signs/symptoms of, 44–45
surgical management of, 60
types of, 41
visual acuity influenced by, 134
glycosylation
in diabetic retinopathy, 68
of lens proteins, 30
guide dogs, 170–171

Healthfinder, 178–179
Health Professionals Follow-Up Study, 92
Healthy People 2010, 110
hearing impairments, 144–145, 151
Heine, C., 125
Holmes, T. H., 113
home care, nursing care, 141–142
Horowitz, A., 120
HTN. *See* hypertension
hyperglycemia
and diabetic retinopathy, 68
tissue damage caused by, 69
hyperopia (short axial eye length), 44